Eye Motility

Edited by Ivana Mravicic

Published in London, United Kingdom

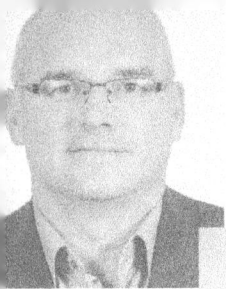
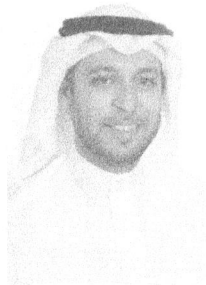
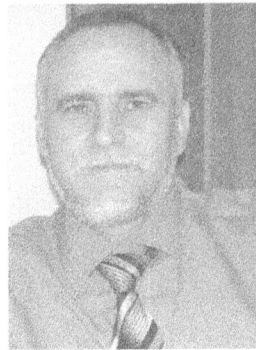
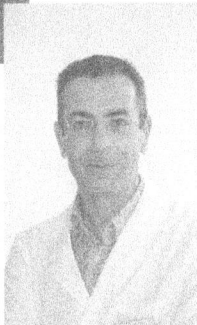
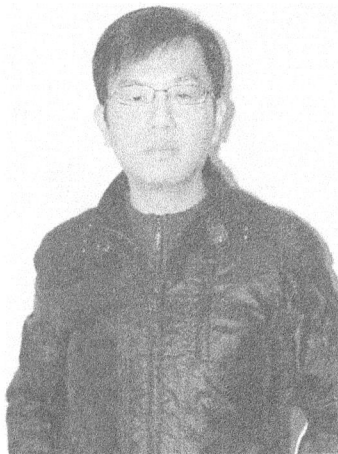
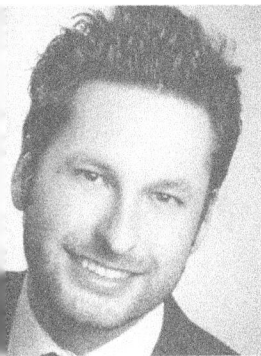
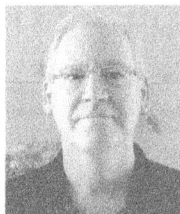

IntechOpen

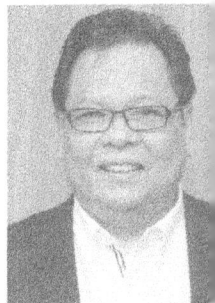
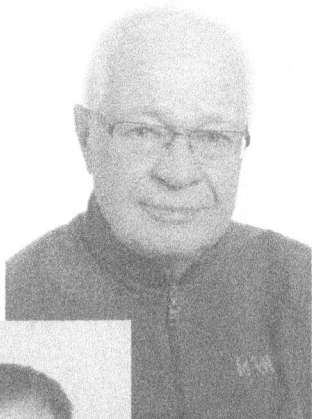
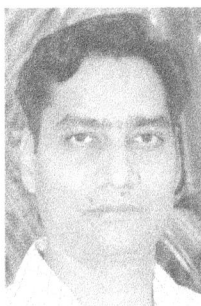
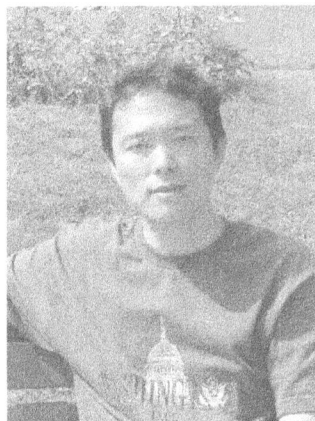
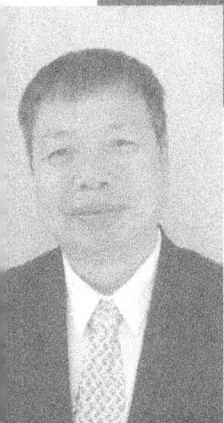
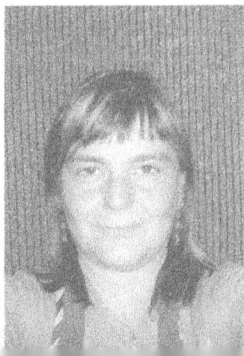

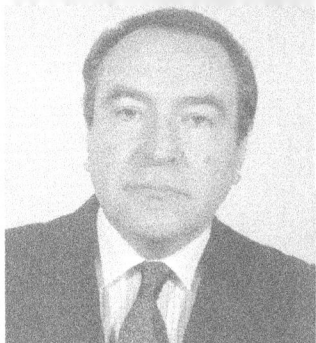

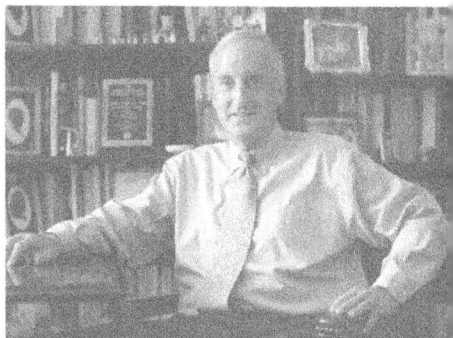

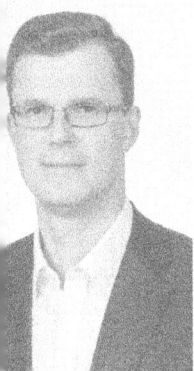

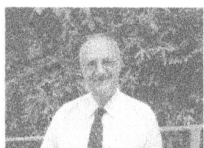

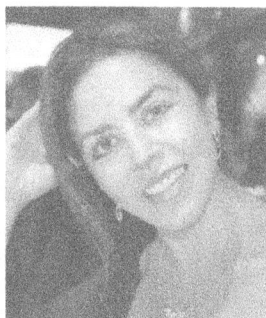

Supporting open minds since 2005

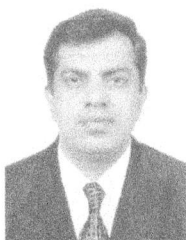

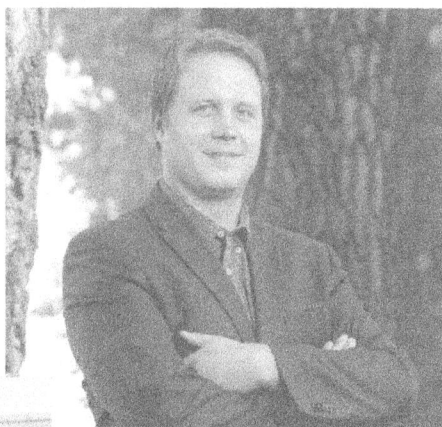

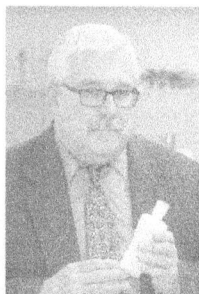

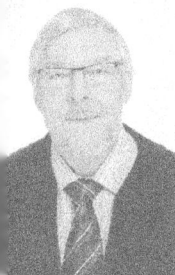

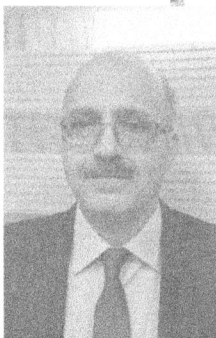

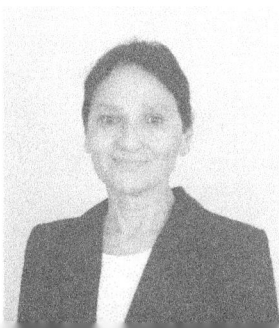

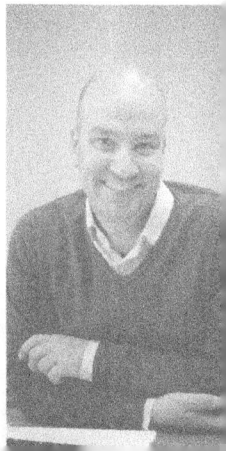

Eye Motility
http://dx.doi.org/10.5772/intechopen.78731
Edited by Ivana Mravicic

Contributors

Roberto Rodriguez-Labrada, Luis Velázquez-Pérez, Yaimeé Vazquez-Mojena, Arvind Morya, Kanchan Solanki, Sahil Bhandari, Anushree Naidu, Kalpit Jangid, Priyanka Rathore, Sujeet Prakash, Sonalika Gogia, Sulabh Sahu, Ivana Mravicic, Maja Bohac, Maja Pauk-Gulic, Vlade Glavota, Selma Lukacevic, Suzana Konjevoda, Ana Didović Pavičić, Samir Čanović, Neda Striber

Notice

Statements and opinions expressed in the chapters are these of the individual contributors and not necessarily those of the editors or publisher. No responsibility is accepted for the accuracy of information contained in the published chapters. The publisher assumes no responsibility for any damage or injury to persons or property arising out of the use of any materials, instructions, methods or ideas contained in the book.

First published in London, United Kingdom, 2019 by IntechOpen
IntechOpen is the global imprint of INTECHOPEN LIMITED, registered in England and Wales, registration number: 11086078, The Shard, 25th floor, 32 London Bridge Street London, SE19SG – United Kingdom
Printed in Croatia

British Library Cataloguing-in-Publication Data
A catalogue record for this book is available from the British Library

Additional hard and PDF copies can be obtained from orders@intechopen.com

Eye Motility
Edited by Ivana Mravicic
p. cm.
Print ISBN 978-1-78984-756-7
Online ISBN 978-1-78984-757-4
eBook (PDF) ISBN 978-1-83881-069-6

We are IntechOpen,
the world's leading publisher of
Open Access books
Built by scientists, for scientists

4,200+
Open access books available

116,000+
International authors and editors

125M+
Downloads

151
Countries delivered to

Our authors are among the

Top 1%
most cited scientists

12.2%
Contributors from top 500 universities

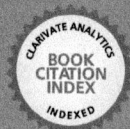

CLARIVATE ANALYTICS
BOOK CITATION INDEX
INDEXED

WEB OF SCIENCE™

Selection of our books indexed in the Book Citation Index
in Web of Science™ Core Collection (BKCI)

Interested in publishing with us?
Contact book.department@intechopen.com

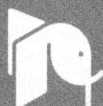

Meet the editor

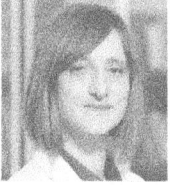

Assistant Professor Ivana Mravicic, MD, graduated from the University of Zagreb Medical School, Croatia, where she completed her MSc and PhD studies. She further developed her clinical and scientific skills with practical training in Munich, Zurich, Tubingen and Hamburg. Dr. Mravicic's field of interest is paediatric ophthalmology and strabismus. She has actively participated at more than 150 international conferences, published many scientific papers and authored and co-authored several books and textbooks. Currently, she is head of the Pediatric Ophthalmology and Strabismus Department at the University Eye Clinic Svjetlost. She also teaches ophthalmology at the University of Rijeka Medical School, Croatia.

Contents

Preface

Having two eyes located at different positions on the head gives humans the ability to perceive two slightly different images (binocularity) that the brain then unites into a single three-dimensional picture (stereo vision). This is a complicated process with many motor and sensory steps that requires our eyes to be perfectly tuned and to work together. This book explains the visual process as well as possible disturbances and consequences that can occur.

Chapter 1 describes visual processing and its associated steps, namely, simultaneous perception, fusion and stereopsis. It explains all steps in detail as well as the tests used to assess them. The chapter also discusses possible disruptions to the process and their consequences.

Chapter 2 pays special attention to the development of children's vision. The development of binocular functions in a child's eyes starts as early as 6 weeks and ends during the first several years of life. Any disruptions can permanently damage this process and may result in the inability to perceive three-dimensional images later in life. The chapter also discusses child eye examinations.

Chapter 3 focuses on nystagmus, which can arise from disruptions at any part of the system that connects the eyes and the brain. Although some kinds of nystagmus are physiological, some pathological types belong to the field of ophthalmology, while others belong to neurology. The chapter makes the distinction between types of nystagmus and explains treatments for "ophthalmological types."

Chapter 4 is dedicated to neurological conditions. Some conditions develop in the places in the brain that are part of the oculomotor as well as the sensory functions of the eyes. The chapter also discusses specific eye movement deficits as well as specific sensory defects.

I would like to thank to my boss Professor Nikica Gabrić, who encouraged me to pursue my professional interest in ophthalmology, and my friend Professor Iva Dekaris for her support. For my love for strabismus and paediatric ophthalmology, I would like to thank Professors Oliver Ehrt and Klaus Peter Boergen.

Ivana Mravicic
Eye Clinic Svjetlost,
Medical School University of Rijeka,
Croatia

Section 1

Introduction

Chapter 1

Introductory Chapter: Why Is Eye Motility Important?

Ivana Mravicic

1. Introduction

Our vision starts with our eyes but the final image that we use in our lives is formed in the brain. Since we have two eyes, we are constantly receiving two different pictures from each eye, respectively. The eyes have to be perfectly tuned together to enable the brain to use two different images and form one three-dimensional picture. The correspondence between the two eyes has to work on several important levels [1].

Correspondence of the two eyes starts at the motor level, which enables the eyes to move in perfect synchrony. Our eyes move with the help of six extraocular muscles: inferior, superior, lateral and medial recti, as well as two oblique muscles named superior and inferior oblique muscles. Because of different insertions of the muscle on the globe, their actions can vary depending on the position of the eye. We can say that the muscles are actually rotating the eye, which results in the possibility of movements in all directions. Muscles are innervated by three cranial nerves (oculomotor, trochlear and abducens). It is impossible to move one eye without the other following. See whether you can do that! When one muscle is innervated, the yoke muscle has the same impulse but in the opposite direction. That synchrony enables our eyes to follow the movement of the other eye.

Perceiving two slightly different images at the same time is called simultaneous perception. When our brain starts to perceive two different pictures as one image, that process is called sensory fusion. To keep sensory fusion working, we need motor fusion that will keep the object in the centre of fovea of each eye. The final ability of the brain is to form one three-dimensional image from two slightly different images that will give us the feeling of depth in space. The final formation of image takes place in the cortex, which plays an important role since more than 50% of cortex is visual cortex [2, 3].

If the synchrony is disrupted, two images are formed in the brain. A disruption can occur at the very beginning in the afferent visual pathway, caused by amblyopia or uncorrected refractive error. In that case, images are too different to be united into one picture. The reason can be in the muscles, caused by inflammation, or autoimmune diseases (Graves' disease) [4]. Muscles are innervated by nerves that travel a long way from their nuclei in the pons and medulla oblongata and are sensitive to traumas of the head or vascular changes. In adult patients, two images result in double vision while, on the other hand, a child's brain has the possibility to adapt and supress one image, which if not recognised can lead to amblyopia of the supressed eye.

Children are a very sensitive group of patients and treating kids bears bigger responsibility than treating adult patients because the child's eye is developing, and unrecognised problem or one which is not treated in the right way can cause serious dysfunction of vision, which is sometimes impossible to fix later. The most sensitive period of visual development is during the first 4 years of life, extending to the age of 7 years. After that age, the sensory system of the brain is formed and improvements are no longer possible [5, 6]. The assessment of children's vision requires special skills, has specific rules and has to be adapted to the age of the child.

Nystagmus is a puzzling, involuntary, rhythmical movement of the eyes. These movements can be caused by some kind of a disruption of the visual development of the child or in the adult age it is often a result of neurological disorders. Our responsibility as ophthalmologists is to recognise which kind of nystagmus is ophthalmological in origin and needs our treatment to encourage visual development. Together with visual aids and some medications, there is some development in new treatments such as biofeedback (making the patients aware of the eye bobbling by sound or touch and, by that, teaching the patient to control nystagmus). On the other hand, neurological nystagmus can be life-threatening and requires urgent neurological examination. Most important signs that have to alarm us to proceed with neurological examination in both children and grown-ups are: the onset of nystagmus after the age of 3 months, oscillopsia (sense of objects moving around us), dissociated and disconjugate nystagmus or associated neurological symptoms (vertigo, nausea, headache, vomiting) [7].

In our work, it is important to be aware of the connection between the eye movement and neurodegenerative diseases since these groups of diseases are becoming more and more common. Neurodegenerative process involves distinct neuron populations in the brain that are involved in circuits of eye movements. The clinical assessment and electrophysiological measurement of the oculomotor function can be useful for understanding the physiopathology and progression of the disease [8].

In conclusion, treating disorders of eye motility is an interesting and demanding process that requires collaboration between different specialities. Ophthalmology and neurology have to work in close collaboration. Another important challenge is treating children whose dynamic of the vision development is very sensitive and specific. Finally, we have a responsibility and the honour to enable and preserve the final perfection of vision which enables us to see the world in different three-dimensional way.

Author details

Ivana Mravicic
Eye Clinic Svjetlost, Medical School University of Rijeka, Croatia

*Address all correspondence to: ivana.mravicic@svjetlost.hr

IntechOpen

References

[1] Von Noorden GK, Campos EC. Binocular Vision and Ocular Motility: Theory and Management of Strabismus. 6th ed, St Louis: Mosby; 2002

[2] Braddick O, Atkinson J. Development of human visual function. Vision Reaserch. 2011;**51**:1588-1609

[3] Khanna, SB, Snyder AC, Smith MA. DOI: 10.1523/JNeurosci.2329-18.2019. E-pub

[4] Pichard T, Paillard A, Santallier M, Criniere L, Pierre P, Pissela PJ, Laure B, Arsene S. Surgical management of strabismus in dysthyroid orbithopathy: A retrospective single-center study of 32 cases. 2108;**41**(8):687-695

[5] Holmes JM, Clarke MP. Amblyopia. The Lancet. 2006;**367**:1343-1351

[6] Grant S, Suttle C, Melmoth DR, Conway ML, Sloper JJ. Age and stereovision-dependent eye-hand coordination deficits in children with amblyopia and abnormal binocularity. Investigative Ophthalmology & Visual Science. 2014;**55**:5687-5701

[7] Ehrt O. Infantile and acquired nystagmus in childhood. Europian Journal Paediatric Neurology. 2012;**6**:567-572

[8] Parvizi J, Van Hoesen GW, Damasio A. The selective vulnerability of brainstem nuclei to Alzheimer's disease. Annals of Neurology. 2001;**49**:53-66

Section 2

Normal Functions of the Eye Motility System

Chapter 2

Binocular Functions

Arvind Kumar Morya, Kanchan Solanki, Sahil Bhandari and Anushree Naidu

Abstract

Binocular single vision is the ability to use both eyes simultaneously so that each eye contributes to a common single perception. Normal binocular single vision occurs with bifoveal fixation and normal retinal correspondence in everyday sight. There are various anatomical and physiological factors concerned in the development of Binocular vision. The development of binocular function starts at 6 weeks and is completed by 6 months. Any obstacles, sensory, motor, or central, in the flex pathway is likely to hamper the development of binocular vision. The presence of these obstacles gives rise to various sensory adaptations to binocular dysfunction. Clinically the tests used can be based on either of the two principles: (A) assessment of relationship between the fovea of the fixing eye and the retinal area stimulated in the squinting eye, viz. Bagolini striated glasses test, red filter test, synoptophore using SMP slides for measuring the objective and subjective angles, and Worth 4-dot test; and (B) Assessment of the visual directions of the two foveae, viz. after image test (Hering Bielschowsky); and Cuppers binocular visuoscopy test (foveo-foveal test of Cuppers). Anomalies of binocular vision results in confusion, diplopia, which leads to suppression, eccentric fixation, anomalous retinal correspondence, and amblyopia.

Keywords: accommodation, binocular vision, stereopsis

1. Introduction

Binocular single vision is the ability of both eyes to contribute to simultaneous perception by contemporaneous use of each of them. Normal binocular single vision results due to the presence of bifoveal fixation and normal retinal correspondence and vice versa. Romano and Romano described binocular vision as—state of simultaneous vision with two seeing eyes that occurs when an individual fixes his visual attention on an object of regard.

Historically, there are two schools of thought with regard to the origin and development of normal binocular vision and spatial orientation.

1. **Theory of empiricism:** This theory describes that binocular vision depends on ontogenetic development. One describes that humans are born without binocularity or spatial orientation and these functions are acquired as a result of experiences from everyday life. This acquisition of this function is aided by all other sensations especially kinesthetic sense.

2. **Theory of nativistic teaching:** This theory states that simultaneous perception and binocular vision occur as result of innate process viz. anatomicophysiological arrangement of components of visual system. This describes that binocular vision is acquired phylogenetically and not ontogenetically [1]. In simple words empiricism states that binocular function develop due to self- learning with trial and error and nativistic theory states that binocular function develops due to coordinated effort of the visual pathway.

2. Binocular vision and its development

During the **initial few years of life** certain normal anatomical and physiological conditions are required for the development of binocular vision [2]. The **factors required** for the development of Binocular vision and which enable the eyes to function in a coordinated manner are as follows [3, 4]

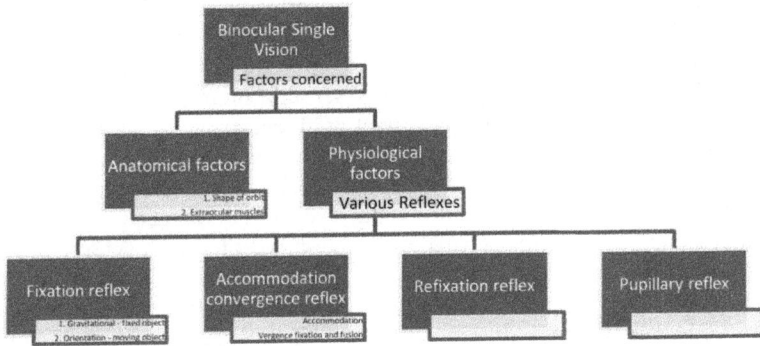

A. **Anatomical factors:** The eyes are spruced up in the orbit in such a way that the visual axis of both eyes is aligned. This occurs as a result of multiple anatomical factors viz.

i. Architecture of the orbit

ii. Ligaments, muscles and connective tissues, i.e., adjacent ocular structures.

The extra-ocular muscles play an important role as they provide motor correspondence because of the reciprocal innervation of the extra-ocular muscles [4].

Following are the aims of motor correspondence:

i. To convert field of vision into field of fixation thereby widening the view.

ii. To ensure that the object of attention is sustained and maintained on fovea.

iii. To ensure that both the eyes are aligned at all times.

B. **Physiological factors:** Normal physiological binocular reflexes determine the development of binocular vision. These physiologic reflexes can be either innate or acquired as a result of appropriate environmental stimulation. Different physiological binocular reflexes are described as below:

i. **Fixation reflexes**

a. *Gravitational reflex, i.e., compensatory fixation reflex:* Whenever there is a movement of body, limbs, etc., this reflex helps maintaining the position of eyes in such a way that the eyes look in the compensating direction to the movement. This reflex occurs as a result of frontal position of eyes as well as utricle and saccule presiding over the tone of vertical rectii and obliques respectively.

b. *Orientation fixation reflex:* A slow continuous movement of eyes can be demonstrated while observing a moving object or a panorama maintaining continuous fixation as opposed to a jerky movement.

ii. **Accommodation convergence reflex:** The aim of this reflex to align the eyes in such a way that the fixation on the object of interest is maintained. It includes three reflexes, viz., (a) vergence fixation reflex, (b) accommodation reflex, and (c) fusional vergence reflex.

iii. **The refixation reflex:** The aim of this reflex is to bring the eye back to the original orientation point or to the new orientation point.

iv. **The pupillary reflex**

3. Fusion reflex, i.e., psycho-optical reflex and its development

Cerebral activity maintains the fusional reflex which are either conditioned or acquired. They develop as a result of experience gained from environmental stimulus. Once these reflexes are formed as a result of continuous reinforcement they transform into unconditioned reflexes. Aimed to form binocular single vision, it consists of all the activities generated from the retina through the brain to maintain the images received on the fovea of both the eyes.

The *elements of fusion mechanism* are:

i. Fixation reflex

ii. Refixation reflex

iii. Conjugate fusional reflexes: the alignment of the two eyes in all positions of gaze is maintained by this reflex.

iv. Disconjugative reflexes: this includes convergence and divergence reflexes.

At birth, the child has random, nonconjugate and aimless ocular movements and the fixation reflex is very poorly developed. During the first few weeks of life there are no pursuit movements. The optomotor reflex is essentially a postnatal event, and it follows the following time schedule:

- First 2–3 weeks—follows light uniocularly

- 6 weeks to 6 months—follows light binocularly

- Convergence reflex is absent at birth. It starts developing during the first month of age and is well developed by 6 months of life.

- The accommodation lags behind the development of convergence due to the delay in the development of ciliary muscles, it develops by 6 months of age.

Various electrophysiological studies have been done in infants, which be proved to be promising in detection of stereoacuity between the age of 2–5 months. But from the age of 6 months to 3 years when the child can sufficiently comprehend to subjects the knowledge about the development of stereoacuity is miniscule. However, it was found that there stereoacuity improves gradually up to the age of 9 years. From the above literature, it is noticed that the sensitive period of development of binocular vision in human beings begins at about 4 months of age, peaks at 2 years, it is well developed by 4 years of age and slowly stops by 9 years of age. Hence it was found that the first 2 years of life is very critical for the development of binocular single vision and any obstacle during the first 2 years can hamper the development of binocular vision. The obstacle in the reflex pathway is likely to hamper the development of binocular vision can be due to the following reasons.

There can be many forms of obstacle in the development of binocular vision viz.

1. Central obstacles

2. Sensory obstacles

- Dioptric obstacles—e.g., opacities in the media, refractive errors that are uncorrected.

- Prolonged uniocular activity—e.g., severe ptosis, anisometropia

- Retinoneural obstacles—lesions of retina, optic nerve

- Proprioceptive obstacle

3. Motor obstacles

- Congenital craniofacial malformations

- CNS lesions—involving the nerve trunks, root of nuclei

The presence of any of these obstacles gives rise to various sensory adaptations to binocular dysfunction disruptive factor is present in the sensitive period. This can be in the form of:

1. Anamolous retinal correspondence

2. Suppression

3. Amblyopia

4. Theories of binocular vision

Projection theory	• Abandoned • Bicentric projection
Isomorphism	• Rigid retinocortical relationship • Gennari's strip an anatomical counterpart of Horopter
Correspondance and Disparity	• Highly accepted one • One to one retinocortical relation • Binocular rivalry
Neurophysiological theory and stereopsis	• Retinogeniculate Striate pathway • Corresponding points and equal receptive fields • Retinal field disparity

4.1 Projection theory of binocular vision

This is an obsolete theory. According to this theory Visual stimuli are exteriorized along the lines of direction. If a person fixates binocularly, a "bicentric" projection is supposed to occur that places the impression of each eye at the point of intersection of the lines of projection [5, 6].

This theory fails to explain certain fundamental observations such as

1. Physiologic diplopia

2. The discrepancies between stimulus distribution and perception

3. Fails completely when interpretation of the sensory phenomena observed in strabismus is attempted.

The basic reason for the failure of the projection theory is that the distinction between physical and subjective space is disregarded and it does not explain the localization to a dioptic-geometric scheme.

4.2 Theory of isomorphism

This theory of binocular vision was developed by Linksz based on a rigid retinocortical relationship [7]. He believed that fusion is based on neuroanatomical connections in the cerebral cortex. The retinas of both the eyes are excited into close proximity within the visual cortex. The corresponding elements are consummated in Gennari's stripe, which he considered to be the anatomical counterpart of the horopter plane in objective space and of the nuclear plane in subjective space. But till date there is no evidence for the physiologic rigidity of the retinocortical relationship or the convergence of the pathways on which it is based.

4.3 Correspondence and disparity theory

According to this theory sensory binocular cooperation is based on system of correspondence and disparity [8]. It assumes the presence of one to one retinocortical relationship between the two eyes. They transmit single visual impression with no depth quality when stimulated simultaneously by one object point. Binocular rivalry occurs when stimulated simultaneously by two object points that differ in character. Diplopia occurs when disparate elements are stimulated by one object point. However, a single visual impression is elicited with depth perception, if horizontal disparity remains within limits of Panum's area. With the increasing disparity the perceived depth increases. However, quality of stereopsis decreases with increasing disparity which may eventually lead to diplopia.

4.4 Neurophysiological theory of binocular vision and stereopsis

Approximately [9] 80% of the neurons in the striate cortex can be stimulated from either eye in response to a visual stimulus, assuming there is a precise and orderly arrangement of connections along the retino-geniculate striate pathway. Of these 75% represented graded response from either left or right eye while 25% are binocularly driven cells and are equally stimulated from each eye. These 75% cells that could be driven by stimulation of either eye had receptive fields of nearly equal size and in corresponding positions of visual field. In normal binocular single vision, optical stimulus will excite a cortical cell only. Only one object feature is detected by each cortical cell and assigned by it to a single locus in space although two receptive fields are involved. Anatomically identical regions in the two retinas are not always occupied by the two receptive fields. There are cells whose fields have exactly corresponding points in the two retina and cells whose fields have slightly different position in the two eyes is seen at a given locus in the retino-optic cortical map. This retinal field disparity is detected by sensitive binocular neurons giving rise to binocular vision and stereopsis which occurs as a result of the difference in direction or distance of the fields in each retina forms the basis of Panum's fusion area.

5. Review of literature

1. Alhagen on binocular vision: In his book of optics, Allahgen followed Gallen in explaining that we have two eyes so that when one is harmed other remains intact and he added that two eyes beautify the face. He clearly described the concept of corresponding points in the image planes of two eyes. He stated that the eyes always move together and by an equal amount, so that visual axis converges on the objective of interest. He then discussed double images produced by an object nearer or farther away than the fixation point, with both the object and fixation point in median plane. He explained that two lines appear in the center because they lie on the visual axis therefore share a common visual direction in the fused image. Allahgen's—center is now called—egocentre and—common axis is called—cyclopean axis.

2. Aguilonius introduced the term—horopter to describe the locus in space within which both fused and diplopic image appear to lie.

3. Veith used the same Euclidean theorems to prove that theoretically the locus of equal angles of binocular subtense is the locus of fused image and both are a circle passing through the center of eyes.

4. In seventeenth and eighteenth century, clearly stated that binocular vision contributes to impression of visual depth.

5. First to specify clearly the geometry of corresponding points and horizontal horopter as the locus of object produced fused images

6. Wheatstone demonstrated the relationship between binocular disparity and depth perception.

7. Stereopsis depends on the registration of disparities but argued that the coincidence of localization of the corresponding pictures received from the two eyes depends on the power of measuring distances of sight which we gain with experience.

8. Inputs from the corresponding regions from two retinas converged on what he called isodynamic cells and that his mechanism forms the basis of unified binocular vision

6. Fusion, diplopia, and the law of sensory correspondence

An object is positioned at a convenient distance in front of an observer at eye level and in the midplane of the head. An image will be received on matching areas of the two retinas if the eyes are properly aligned and if the object is fixated binocularly. The two images will be the same in size, illuminance, and color if both eyes are functioning normally and equally. Though two separate physical (retinal) images are formed, only one visual object is perceived by the observer. This phenomenon is so natural to us that the naive observer believes it to be normal, he is surprised only if he sees double. Yet the opposite—single binocular vision from two distinct retinal images—is the truly remarkable phenomenon that needs an explanation.

Binocular single vision occurs when the image formed in the retina from each eye contributes to a single, common perception. It is considered in three grades:

- **Sensory:** It is the ability to perceive an image formed from each eye simultaneously.

- **Motor:** It is the ability of both the eyes to maintain sensory fusion through a range vergence movements.

- **Stereopsis:** It is the perception of depth based on binocular disparity.

7. Prerequisites for binocular vision

1. Central fixation with normal visual acuity

2. Accurate oculomotor control-bifoveal fixation

3. Normal inter retinal correspondence of visual directions

4. Sensory mechanism to provide haplopia

5. Neural mechanisms to extract selective depth signals

Binocular single vision can be classified into three stages according to Worth's classification (**Figure 1**)

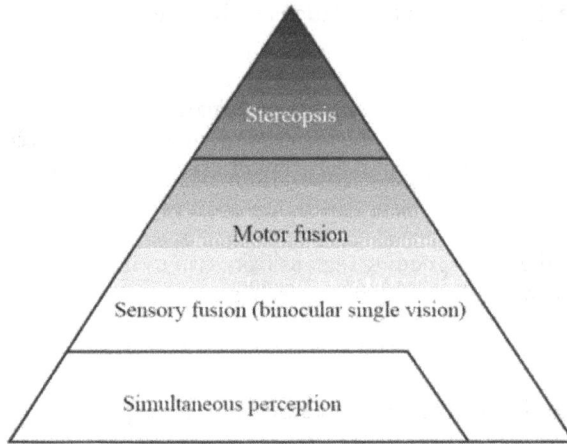

Figure 1.
The classical model of binocular visual function is composed of three hierarchical degrees.

1. Simultaneous perception and superimposition

2. Fusion

3. Stereoscopic vision

7.1 Simultaneous perception and superimposition

The ability of both the eyes to perceive simultaneously two images, one formed on each retina is defined as simultaneous perception. Simultaneous perception of the two images formed on corresponding areas, with the projection of these images to the same position in space is superimposition. This occurs based on the correspondence whether it is normal or abnormal. If fusion does not occur then two similar images are seen as separate but superimposed and no fusion range can be demonstrated.

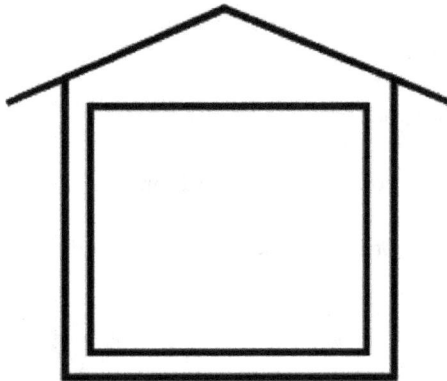

Image 1.
Simultaneous perception—image for the first eye.

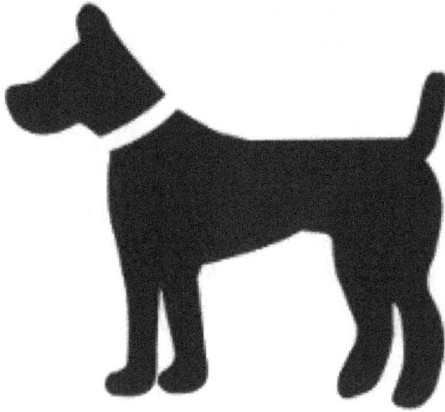

Image 2.
Simultaneous perception—image for second eye.

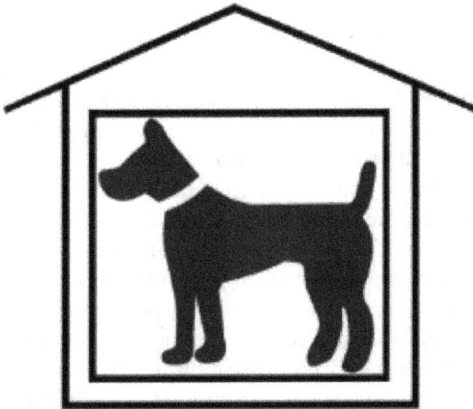

Image 3.
Simultaneous perception—binocular vision image.

Exemplary on **Image 1** there is element visible for one eye and on **Image 2** visible for second eye. Patient with ability to simultaneous perception should perceive image similar to **Image 3**.

7.2 Fusion

Fusion is defined as the unification of visual excitations from the corresponding retinal images into a single visual perception. Fusion can be either sensory or motor.

7.2.1 Sensory fusion

The hallmark of retinal correspondence is the sensory fusion which is defined as is the ability of both the eyes to perceive two similar images, one formed on each retina, when interpreted as one single visual image. The images not only must be located on corresponding retinal areas but also should be sufficiently similar with respect to size, brightness and sharpness to permit sensory are the prerequisites for sensory fusion. A severe obstacle to fusion are unequal images.

7.2.2 Motor fusion

The ability to align both the eyes in such a way that sensory fusion can be maintained is termed as Motor fusion. Retinal disparity formed outside Panum's area and the eyes moving in opposite direction which may be horizontal, vertical or cyclovergence is the stimulus for these fusional eye movements. Unlike sensory fusion, motor fusion is a function of the extrafoveal retinal periphery. Fusion, whether sensory or motor, is always a central process, i.e., it takes place in the visual cortex.

7.3 Stereopsis

The fused image will be perceived in vivid depth nearer or farther to the point of fixation within some range of limiting conditions, when two similar images are presented to both the eyes with a binocular disparity that has a horizontal component. The objects give rise to the stereoscopic depth from Horizontal binocular disparities, e.g., arrow at different distances and it gives rise to stereoscopic depth perception. Here the arrowhead has a lesser eccentricity on the nasal retina of the right eye than on the temporal retina of the left eye. The fovea is the site of fixation. The observer is aware alternately of the image to one eye and the image to the other if such dichoptic image formed is of high contrast, due to binocular rivalry that forms between the two monocular images. As a result of interocular suppression if one eye is strongly dominant as a result of either stimulus characteristics or organismic variables, perception of the image in the other eye may be entirely absent. Prolonged periods of dichoptic summation may be obtained, during which the different stimuli in the two eyes appear to be summed together as if their contrasts were added linearly throughout the dichoptic field. If however, the stimulus contrast is low for dichoptic stimuli. When the presentation time is brief (150 ms) dichoptic summation also is obtained for high contrast stimuli.

Where the image appears doubled but clearly at a different depth from zero-disparity targets stereoscopic depth from horizontal disparities is perceived both in the region of binocular fusion of the monocular targets into a single image and also in the region of diplopia, the smallest disparity interval that produces reliable depth discrimination under particular conditions is stereo acuity.

8. Sensory adaptations in binocular vision

8.1 Suppression

Suppression is a neuro-physiological phenomenon of the eye to prevent diplopia and confusion by suppressing the non-dominant image at the cortical level. Diplopia occurs when fovea of one eye and extra foveal point of the other eye is stimulated simultaneously. Confusion occurs when dissimilar image is projected on fovea of both the eyes.

8.1.1 Types of suppression

Facultative suppression: In Facultative suppression visual acuity is not affected under monocular conditions. Facultative suppression occurs only under binocular conditions.

Obligatory suppression: It occurs even under monocular conditions resulting in diminished visual acuity which further leads to amblyopia.

Central and peripheral suppression: To avoid confusion foveal image of the deviating eye is suppressed which is known as central suppression. Similarly to avoid diplopia extra foveal image of the deviating eye is suppressed resulting in peripheral suppression.

Monocular or alternating: Monocular suppression occurs when the image from the dominant eye always predominates over the image from the deviating eye, so that the image from the latter is constantly suppressed. This leads to amblyopia. When suppression alternates between the two eyes amblyopia is less likely to occur.

8.2 Anamolous retinal correspondence

Anamolous retinal correspondence is a type of sensory adaptation in which fovea of one eye shares a common visual direction with the extra foveal point of the other eye. This is an adaptation in manifest squint resulting in binocular single vision. It is known as anomalous because extra foveal point of one eye corresponds to foveal point of the other eye. But in contrast to eccentric fixation under monocular conditions, fovea of deviating eye takes the fixation which forms the basis for cover test.

Prerequisites for anomalous retinal correspondence:

1. Small angle of deviation

2. Constant deviation

3. Extra foveal point should be close to the fovea

8.3 Motor adaptations to strabismus

Motor adaptation is in the form of abnormal head posture and occurs primarily in children with congenitally abnormal eye movements who use the abnormal head posture to maintain the binocular single vision.

9. Retinal correspondence

Retinal correspondence occurs when the retinal points of both the eyes share a common visual direction. Non corresponding retinal points will never have a common visual direction.

9.1 Types of retinal correspondence

9.1.1 Normal retinal correspondence

Normal retinal correspondence is defined when fovea of one eye corresponds to the fovea of the other eye and they both share a common visual direction. In NRC, points located nasal to the fovea in one eye correspond to the points located temporal to the fovea of the other eye.

9.1.2 Abnormal retinal correspondence

Anamolous retinal correspondence is a type of sensory adaptation in which fovea of one eye shares a common visual direction with the extra foveal point of the other eye. This is an adaptation in manifest squint resulting in binocular single vision. It is known as anomalous because extra foveal point of one eye corresponds to foveal point of the other eye. But in contrast to eccentric fixation under monocular conditions, fovea of deviating eye takes the fixation which forms the basis for cover test.

Prerequisites for anomalous retinal correspondence:

1. Small angle of deviation

2. Constant deviation

3. Extra foveal point should be close to the fovea.

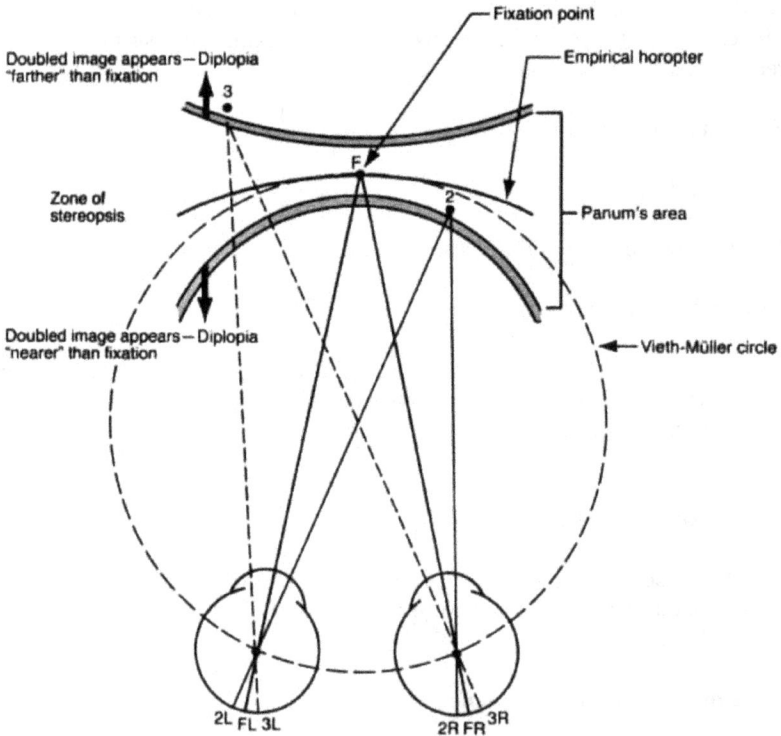

Figure 2.
Empirical horopter. F, fixation point; FL and FR, left and right foveae, respectively. Point 2, falling within Panum's area, is seen singly and stereoscopically. Point 3 falls outside Panum's area and is therefore seen doubly.

10. Concept of a Horopter

The term Horopter (**Figure 2**) is derived from Greek words, horos-boundary, opter-observer, was first introduced in 1613 by Aguilonius [5]. The horopter is a curved line formed when all the corresponding points are projected in space at a particular distance from the observer. Hence it is the locus of all points in the space that stimulates the corresponding points of the retina leading to a binocular single vision.

Geometric Vieth Muller horopter is a theoretical horopter. It is a geometrically constructed circle which passes through the corresponding points of the two eyes. But actually it is not spherical, it is flatter. The actual—**Empirical horopter** curve also known as the longitudinal horopter is slightly flatter than Vieth Muller Geometric horopter. It is formed by using longitudinal bars positioned such that they appear equidistant. The difference between the geometric and the empirical horopter is known as the Hering-Hillebrand deviation. Very small areas around the corresponding points can be binocularly fused to see singly. This is known as Panum's area of binocular fusion. Diplopia elicited by an object point off the horopter but within Panum's fusional area is known as physiological diplopia. Panum's area is narrowest at fovea (6–10° of arc) and broader in periphery (30–40° of arc). Objects lying outside the Panum's area will be perceived double when viewed binocularly. Even though the fusion occurs, a perceptual effort is made which is appreciated by the cortex as depth perception. So Panum's area is physiological basis for our depth perception.

11. Stereopsis (Figure 3)

It is the ability of both the eyes to fuse images that lie within Panum's fusional area resulting in three dimensional perception of the object. Diplopia elicited by an object point off the horopter but within Panum's fusional area is known as physiological diplopia. Images of a single object that do not stimulate corresponding retinal points in both eyes are said to be disparate; binocular disparity is defined as the difference in position of corresponding points between images in the two eyes.

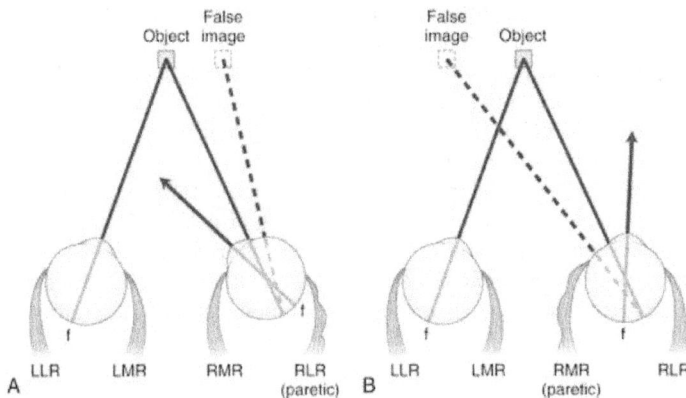

Figure 3.
Crossed and uncrossed disparities result when objects produce images that are formed on closely separated retinal points. Any point within Panum's area yields a percept of a single image, while points outside Panum's area produces diplopia.

Binocular disparity or Physiological diplopia can be of two types crossed (temporal or heteronymous) and uncrossed (nasal or homonymous). Crossed diplopia occurs when objects lie in front of the horopter. In crossed diplopia the monocular image of the object perceived by the right eye is displaced to left and the image perceived by the left eye is displaced to the right. Uncrossed diplopia occurs when objects lie behind the horopter. Hence in uncrossed diplopia the monocular image of the object perceived by the right eye is displaced to the right and the image perceived by the left eye is displaced to the left (**Figure 3**).

12. Stereoscopic acuity

It can be defined as the disparity beyond which no stereoscopic effect can be produced. A threshold of 15–30 arc seconds is considered excellent; however, there is no standardization for the same. There is a critical distance calculated to be 150–200 m beyond which the stereopsis does not work as there is a threshold for stereopsis. The threshold of stereoscopic acuity also depends on the motion of both eye as well as the target object. For static targets the stereoacuity ranges from 2 to 10 arc sec which increases to 40 arc sec for objects in motion. Stereoacuity is maximal about 0.25° off dead center in the foveola. As we move along the x axis the stereoacuity decreases exponentially. Stereopsis is not present beyond 15° from the center. There is a similar exponential decline in the stereoacuity when the target is moved in front or behind the horopter along the y-axis. Stereopsis although is very essential for spatial orientation, it is not the only means of it. The various monocular clues to spatial orientation can be:

> **Apparent size:** It depends on the size of the object as well as the distance of the object from the retina. The objects that are closer to the retina appear larger in size and those farther away appear smaller. Similarly as the object move towards the retina it appears to be increased in size.
> **Interposition:** The objects that are relatively near conceal the objects that are far.
> **Aerial perspective:** Environmental factors like water vapor, dust and smoke cause scattering of the light and hence cause decrease in the color saturation as well as visibility of the distance object.
> **Shading:** Whenever light falls on a solid object it casts shadow and when it falls on the concave surface the shadow is cast in a graded manner.
> **Geometric perspective:** The line that is parallel pragmatically appears to join together near the horizon, e.g., railroad tracks.
> **Relative velocity:** The velocity of image of a moving target that is at a distance is slower that the velocity of image of a moving target that is near.
> **Motion parallax:** If the fixation point is at an intermediate distance the objects that are nearer to it move in the opposite direction when the head is moved and those that are farther away from the fixation point move along with the head.

13. Fusion

Fusion is defined as the amalgamation of visual impulses from the corresponding retinal images into a single visual percept.

13.1 Sensory fusion

When two similar images are formed on the corresponding areas of each eye, the ability to interpret them as one is termed as sensory fusion. Retinal correspondence can be certified from the fact that a single image is formed. Size, brightness and sharpness of similar degree are equally essential components required for sensory fusion to occur as is the retinal correspondence images of unequal size are a severe obstacle to fusion.

13.2 Motor fusion

For the sensory fusion to be maintained it is essential that the eyes are aligned and the ability to do so is termed as motor fusion. Retinal disparity outside Panum's area and the eyes moving in opposite direction (vergence) are the stimuli for the fusional movements. Motor fusion is the exclusive function of the extrafoveal retinal periphery, unlike sensory fusion which is dependent on fovea. However both sensory and motor fusion are central processes the control of which lies in the visual cortex.

13.3 Diplopia

When there is a simultaneous stimulation of two disparate retinal points by a point object, there occurs perception of the object in two different subjective visual directions. An object point seen simultaneously in two directions appears double. Double vision is the hallmark of retinal disparity.

13.4 Binocular rivalry

Retinal rivalry may be observed when dissimilar contours are presented to corresponding retinal areas and fusion becomes impossible. When areas of retinal correspondence are stimulated by dissimilar object, fusion fails to occur and leads to confusion. To surpass this confusion, image from one of the eyes is suppressed. The constant foveal suppression of one eye leads to complete sensory dominance of the other eye with cessation of rivalry, which is a major obstacle to binocular vision. For binocular vision to be functional presence of retinal rivalry is must.

14. Grades of binocular vision

Worth's classification of binocular vision:

Grade I: Simultaneous perception is the most basic essential prerequisite for binocular single vision. It is the power to see two dissimilar objects simultaneously.

Grade II: It represents true fusion with some amplitude. The two images are not only fused, but some effort is made to maintain this fusion in spite of difficulties. Addition of motor component to the sensory fusion represents second grade of binocular vision.

Grade III: This is the highest grade of binocular vision in which the images are not only fused but also a stereoscopic view of the image is produced. It is the ability to obtain an impression of depth by the superimposition of two pictures of the same object taken from slightly different angles.

Binocular vision assessment:
All the tests are aimed at assessing the presence or absence of:

1	Normal or abnormal retinal correspondence
2	Suppression
3	Simultaneous perception
4	Fusion
5	Stereopsis

It is essential to assess the visual acuity, fixation in the deviating eye and direction and amount of deviation in every case.

Test for retinal correspondence:

Clinically the tests used can be based on either of the two principles:

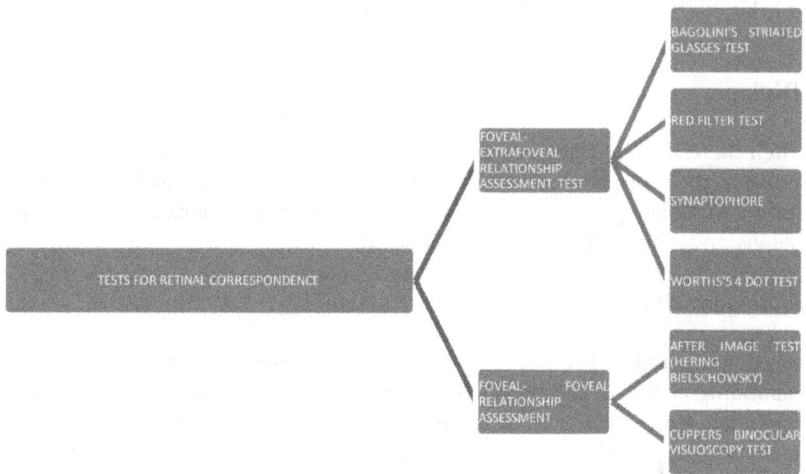

1. **Bagolini striated glasses test:** The patient is asked to fixate a small light, after being provided

With plano lenses with narrow fine striations across one meridian (micro Maddox cylinders) a source of light is seen as a line at right angles to the striations. The axis of striations of the eyes is kept at right angles to each other. The interpretation of this test is as follows:

a. Symmetrical cross response

    i. In the absence of a manifest squint, a cross response indicates a normal bifoveal correspondence (NRC).

    ii. In the presence of a manifest squint, a cross response indicates an anomalous retinal correspondence (ARC) of harmonious type (subjective angle of deviation of zero).

b. Asymmetrical cross response or two lines cutting each other at some other point than midline, indicates an incomitant squint with normal retinal correspondence (diplopia response).

    c. Single line seen: If only one line is seen it indicates suppression of the other eye (suppression response).

    d. Cross response with central gap in one line indicates a central suppression scotoma in that eye.

2. **Red filter test:** It is a characteristic test used to check dissociation between two eye. It is done by placing a red filter over the preferential fixating eye while it fixates over a small light source.

Results can be interpreted as:

    a. *Normal retinal correspondence:* two lights are reported by the patient; one red and other white.

        i. In cases of homonymus (uncrossed) diplopia, patient reports red light to the right of white light when right eye is tested.

        ii. In cases of heterogeneous (crossed) diplopia, patient reports red light to the left of white light when right eye is tested.

    b. *Abnormal retinal correspondence:* It can be of two types:

        i. In cases of harmonious heterophoria patient reports only single light which is pinkish in color because of superimposition of white and red light.

        ii. In unharmonious heterophoria patient reports two different types of light depending on the direction of deviation.

    c. *Suppression:* Patient reports only single light source (more commonly white line). It depends on the degree of dominance of the other eye and the density of the red filter used.

Measurement of angle of anomaly: It is the difference between objective and subjective angle of deviation seen in cases of abnormal retinal correspondence. The angle of anomaly is a measure of the degree of shift in visual direction.

Procedure of estimating the angle of anomaly: This test is done with the help of synaptophore. The SMP slides are used in this test. The position of synaptophore arms is kept at zero. The examiner flashes light behind each slide and keeps on moving the arm till the time there is no further movement (alternate cover test). When there is no further movement the angle of each arm is noted. The sum total of the angles recorded of both the arms is the objective angle of anomaly. The angle at which the visual targets are superimposed is the subjective angle of anomaly.

Objective angle (D): Angle by which the visual axis of eye fails to intersect the target of regard.

Subjective angle (S): Angle between the zero measure of the deviating eye and point in that eye corresponding to the fovea of other eye.

Interpretation:

a. Normal retinal correspondence: D = S; Angle of anomaly is zero.

b. Abnormal retinal correspondence: D is not equal to S.

i. Harmonious ARC: Subjective angle is zero. Angle of anomaly is equal to objective angle.

ii. Unharmonious ARC: Angle of anomaly is less than objective angle.

iii. Paradoxical ARC: Angle of anomaly is greater than objective angle of duration.

3. **Worth 4-dot test:** This is a simple test using the principle of red-green color dissociation. It is more dissociating than the Bagolini's glasses and hence is less physiological. The apparatus for this test consists of a box containing four panes of glass, arranged in diamond formation, which are illuminated internally from a light source. The two internal panes are green, the upper one is red and lower one is white. The patient wears a green lens in front of the right eye, and a red lens in front of the left eye. The test can be performed separately for distance and near vision. The interpretation of this test is as follows:

a. If BSV is present all four lights are seen

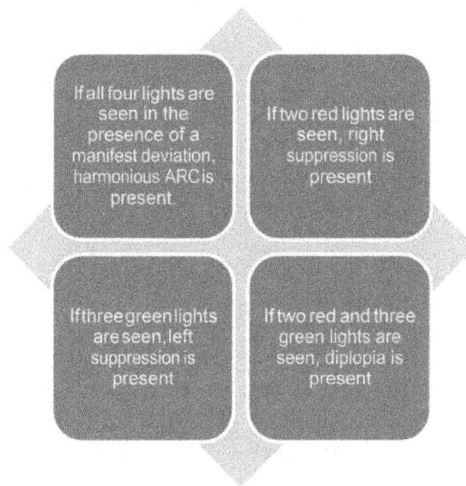

If all four lights are seen in the presence of a manifest deviation, harmonious ARC is present.

If two red lights are seen, right suppression is present

If three green lights are seen, left suppression is present

If two red and three green lights are seen, diplopia is present

b. If the green and red lights alternate, alternating suppression is present.

4. **Hering Bielschowsky after-image test:** This is a highly dissociating orthoptic test in which fovea of the two eyes is flashed with linear afterimage horizontal in right eye and vertical in left eye since each eye is individually stimulated, only the fovea are at the center of the after images.

Procedure: Subject is asked to concentrate on the central black spot of the glowing filament with alternate eye occluding the other eye. The stimulus is first presented to the better eye and then vertically to the opposite eye. This stimulus is presented for 20 s to each eye and then subject is asked to tell the distance between gaps of two images.

a. If central fixation is present, the gaps correspond to the visual direction of each fovea.

Results are as follows:

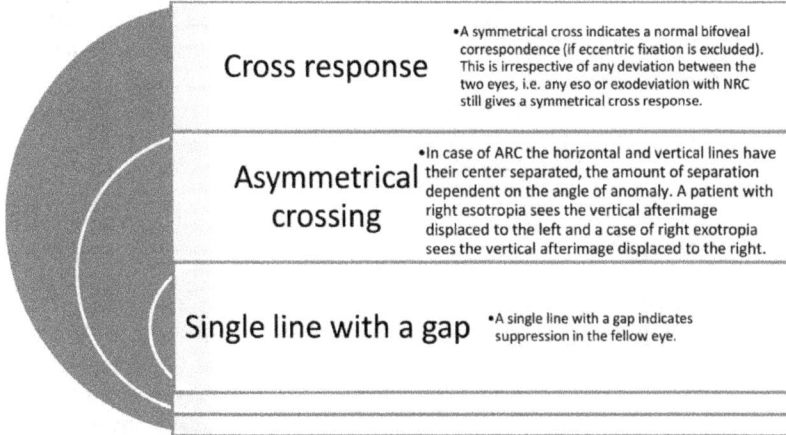

Cross response	• A symmetrical cross indicates a normal bifoveal correspondence (if eccentric fixation is excluded). This is irrespective of any deviation between the two eyes, i.e. any eso or exodeviation with NRC still gives a symmetrical cross response.
Asymmetrical crossing	• In case of ARC the horizontal and vertical lines have their center separated, the amount of separation dependent on the angle of anomaly. A patient with right esotropia sees the vertical afterimage displaced to the left and a case of right exotropia sees the vertical afterimage displaced to the right.
Single line with a gap	• A single line with a gap indicates suppression in the fellow eye.

1. **Foveo-foveal test of cuppers:** This test is done to analyze the angle of anamoly in the presence of eccentric fixation. It determines whether the two foveae have same or different visual directions.

15. Suppression

Suppression involves active inhibition at the visual cortex level when the blurred image from one eye is inhibited under binocular condition. Pre requisite for suppression is large angle deviation, constant deviation and deviation that occurs in early childhood.

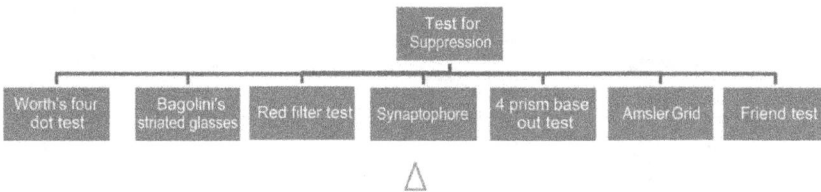

Test for Suppression

Worth's four dot test — Bagolini's striated glasses — Red filter test — Synaptophore — 4 prism base out test — Amsler Grid — Friend test

15.1 Testing extent of suppression

The extent or the area of suppression can be charted under binocular conditions (fixating with one eye while the field of other eye is charted). This may be done by different methods:

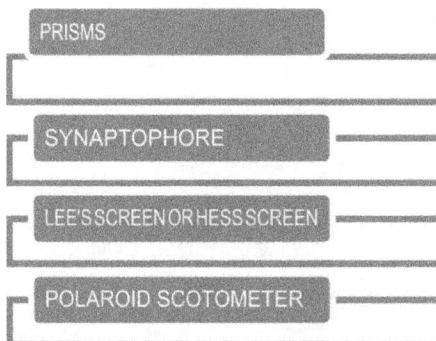

PRISMS

SYNAPTOPHORE

LEE'S SCREEN OR HESS SCREEN

POLAROID SCOTOMETER

The various responses that can be observed are:
More the dissociation larger is the single scotoma in prism's, Lee's.
Lesser the dissociation, 2–3 discrete scotomas are seen, one is foveal scotoma about 2–3° in size and diplopia point scotoma, e.g., Aulhorn phase difference haploscope and Polaroid scotometer.
Depth/intensity of scotoma: Depth of scotoma is determined by Graded Density Filter Bar of Bagolini. In it as the denser filter is applied over dominant eye, the scotoma in amblyopic eye becomes small.

15.2 4 Δ base out prism test

This test is used for diagnosing a small facultative scotoma in a patient with monofixation syndrome and no manifest small deviation. In this test, a 4▲ Base out Prism is placed before one eye and then other under binocular viewing condition
Patient with bifixation show a bilateral version movement away from the eye covered by the Prism followed by unilateral fusional convergence movement of the eye not under the Prism.
In Monofixation no movement is seen when Prism is placed over the nonfixating eye. A refixation version is seen when Prism is placed over fixating eye but then fusional convergence does not occur.

16. Simultaneous macular perception

Simultaneous macular perception occurs when visual signals transferred from the two eyes to the cortex are perceived at the same time. It is the ability to see two dissimilar objects simultaneously. Commonly used synaptophore contain slides such as Bird and Cage, Lion and Cage. The interpretation is as follows:

Simultaneous macular perception	Subtend angle at nodal point
Simultaneous foveal perception slide	1°
Simultaneous parafoveal perception slides	1–3°
Simultaneous paramacular perception slides	3–5°
Simultaneous peripheral perception slides	<5°

The term simultaneous perception does not necessarily mean bifoveal fixation as it can also occur in Anamolous retinal correspondence. It just indicates the presence or absence of suppression.
Normal range of amplitudes of fusion:

Type of vergence		Amplitude range
Horizontal vergence	Convergence	35–40 Δ
	Divergence	5–7 Δ
Verticgence	Supravergence	3 Δ
	Infravergence	3 Δ
Cyclovergence	—	2–3 Δ

It is necessary to assess fusion for both viz. determining the prognosis and outlining the management of the patients of strabismus.

To restore binocular single vision fusion is essential.

Following are the tests used to determine the presence of fusion are:

- Worth 4-dot test

- Bagolini striated glasses

- Synaptophore

Following tests can be used to determine stereopsis: Tests to determine stereopsis are based on two principles viz.

1. The targets used are such that they lie in two planes, but are constructed in such a way that they cause stimulation of disparate retinal elements which gives a three-dimensional effect, for example:

   - Concentric rings, i.e., circular perspective diagrams

   - Titmus fly test

   - TNO test

   - Random dot stereograms

   - Polaroid test

   - Lang's stereo test

   - Stereoscopic targets presented haploscopically in major amblyoscope

2. Using targets that are three dimensional (e.g., Lang's two pencil test)

Tests used to determine stereopsis can be qualitative or quantitative. The unit for measurement of stereopsis is seconds of an arc.

- Following are the qualitative tests for stereopsis:

   - Lang's 2 pencil test

   - Synaptophore

- Following are the quantitative tests for stereopsis:

   - Random dot test

   - TNO Test

   - Lang's stereo test

Polarization can also be used to determine stereopsis: Vectographs and images, used as targets seen by one eye are polarized at 90° using polarized glasses.

- Titmus stereo fly test

- Polaroid test

- Random dot stereograms

- TNO test

16.1 Stereograms

There are two stereograms

1. Both eyes should be used together to see the one with three concentric circles and a check dot for each eye.

2. One with three eccentric circles has to be seen with each eye separately. Interpretation:

    a. Patient sees concentric circles: Stereopsis is present.

    b. Patient sees eccentric circles: Should be asked whether the inner circles are towards right or left. This will help us determine whether the disparate elements are suppressed in right or left eye.

    c. Vectographs: Consists of two targets imprinted on a Polaroid material in such a manner that each target is polarized at 90° with respect to the other. A polarized spectacle is provided to the patient so that each target is seen separately with the two eyes.

A. **Titmus stereo test:** Gross stereoscopic is checked using a stereoscopic pattern representing a housefly. It aids to orient the patient (threshold 3000 s of arc).

    a. *Advantage:* Young children can also perform the test.

    b.*Disadvantage:* Stereopsis using this test is only near stereopsis.

B. **Polaroid test:** There are two types of test that are commonly used

    a. *With animals printed:* It consists of three rows of animals. There one animal in each row which is imaged disparately (threshold 100, 200 and 400 s of arc, respectively). There is also one animal in each row that is printed heavily black which forms the misleading clue. The child is then asked to point out which one of the animals stands out. A child without stereopsis will name the heavily printed animal as the one that stands out.

    b. *With circles:* It consists of nine sets of four circles arranged in the form of a diamond. In this test there are nine sets of four circles which are arranged to form a diamond. One of these circles is imaged dispared in each set randomly. The threshold ranges from 800 to 40 s of arc. The child is asked to push down the circle that stands out. If the stereopsis is limited the child makes mistakes.

C. **E-random dot test:** In this test, there are two cards, one with E printed and the other is blank. The child is explained about the procedure using a test card. After explaining the procedure the child is provided with a polaroid glass and then child is shown the test cards. The child is asked to answer which card has E printed on it.

D. **Random dot stereogram of Julesz:** In this test when the child sees uniocularly, the stereogram reveals random dots scattered everywhere. When viewed binocularly, there appears a square that lies at various depth perception above or below the paper. This exposes child to the requirements similar to that in daily life.

16.2 Binocular vision anomalies

In anamolies of binocular vision there occurs in confusion, diplopia that results in suppression, eccentric fixation, anomalous retinal correspondence and amblyopia.

16.2.1 Classification

Duane's classification forms the basis of classification of anomalies of binocular vision in the field of optometry. This classification system evolved from a four category system to a nine-category system that was developed by Wick. Following parameters are used for classification: (a) distance phoria and (b) AC/A ratio. The accommodative classification system was developed by Donders3 and modified by Duke-Elder and Abrams. Ocular motor dysfunction is a distinct clinical entity in which fixation, pursuit and saccadic anomalies are included. **Table 1** is a summary of the classification system for binocular, accommodative and ocular motor anomalies.

AC/A ratio	Anomalies
Low AC/A ratio	Convergence insufficiency
	Divergence insufficiency
Normal AC/A ratio	Fusional vergence dysfunction
	Basic esophoria
	Basic exophoria
High AC/A ratio	Convergence excess
	Divergence excess
Accommodative anomalies	Accommodative insufficiency
	Ill-sustained accommodation
	Accommodative excess
	Accommodative infacility
Ocular motor anomalies	Ocular motor dysfunction

Table 1.
Summary of the classification system for binocular, accommodative and ocular motor anomalies.

Author details

Arvind Kumar Morya[1*], Kanchan Solanki[2], Sahil Bhandari[2] and Anushree Naidu[2]

1 Department of Ophthalmology, All India Institute of Medical Sciences, Jodhpur, Rajasthan, India

2 Consultant Ophthalmologist and Vitreoretinal Surgeon Guru Hasti Chikitsalya, Jodhpur, Rajasthan, India

*Address all correspondence to: moryaak@aiimsjodhpur.edu.in

IntechOpen

References

[1] Von Noorden GK. In: von Noorden GK, Campos EC, editors. Binocular Vision and Ocular Motility: Theory and Management of Strabismus. 6th ed. United State of America: Mosby Inc.; 1928

[2] Tyler CW. Chap. 24: Binocular vision. In: 0331—Foundations of Clinical Ophthalmology. New York: Lipincott Williams and Wilkins; Vol. 15. pp. 35-55. R2-05-21-04

[3] Kaufman FL, Alm A, Adler FH. Adler's Physiology of Eye: Clinical Application. 10th ed. St Louis: Mosby; 2003

[4] Duane TD, Tasman W, Jaeger EA. Duane's Clinical Ophthalmology. New York: Lippincott Williams & Wilkins; 2005

[5] von Helmholtz H. In: Southhall PC, editor. Helmholtz's Treatise on Physiological Optics. New York: Dover Publications; 1962. English Translation from 3rd German ed.; Ithaca, NY: Optical Society of America; 1924. Quoted from Reprint

[6] Duane A. Binocular vision and projection. Archives of Ophthalmology. 1931;**5**:734

[7] Linksz A. Physiology of the eye. In: Linksz A, editor. Vision. Vol. 2. New York: Grune & Stratton; 1952

[8] Burian HM. Studien u berzweia ugigesTiefensehenbeio rtlicherAbblendung. Graefe's Archive for Clinical and Experimental Ophthalmology. 1936;**136**:172

[9] Hubel DH, Wiesel TN. Receptive fields of single neurons in the cat's striate cortex. Journal of Physiology (London). 1959;**148**:574

Chapter 3

Ophthalmologic Examination of the Child

*Suzana Konjevoda, Neda Striber, Samir Čanović
and Ana Didović Pavičić*

Abstract

The ophthalmologic examination of the child consists of an assessment of the physiological function, anatomic eye, and visual system status. A comprehensive eye examination of the child should include history of presenting problem, patient's and family's medical histories, estimation of fixation and measurement of visual acuity, assessment of binocular vision, Bruckner test, assessment of ocular motility, Hirschberg's test, cover/uncover test, and assessment of anterior and posterior segments. The order of examination may vary depending on the child's cooperation. The record of the child's level of cooperation during the examination is of great benefit in the interpretation of the results.

Keywords: examination, strabismus, child, visual acuity, binocular vision, ophthalmological assessment

1. Introduction

The ophthalmologic examination of the child consists of anamnesis or, in this case, heteroanamnesis, physiological function evaluation, and anatomic eye and visual system status. The record of the level of cooperation of the child with the examination is of great benefit in the interpretation of the results. The order of the examination may vary depending on the level of child's collaboration. The visual acuity test should be done before the fusion break test, as well as the visual acuity and bulbomotor examination before using cycloplegic [1].

Examination should include the following elements:

1. Anamnesis

2. Clinical examination

The following tests are of particular importance when examining a child but are indispensable when there is a strabism. If we do not set suspicion of strabism when we examine the child, we can skip some of the following steps:

- Estimation of fixation and measurement of visual acuity

- Testing of binocularity/stereovision

- Binocular red reflex (Brückner) test

- Motility/versions and vergency

- Hirschberg's test

- Cover/uncover test

- Strabismic angle measurements

- Examination of the anterior eye segment

- Skiascopy

- Fundus examination

There are numerous divisions of strabismus—according to the time of occur-rence, presumed etiology, direction of visual axes, that is, clinical manifestation, frequency, affected eye—only to name some [2]. The simplest is the one dividing the strabismus on congenital and acquired forms. In the former, in the vast majority of cases, the etiology is unknown. Actually, it is not present from the birth on but usually occurs and develops in the first months of life. Therefore it might be better to name them early onset strabismus than congenital [3].

On the contrary, acquired strabismus occurs later, and usually the cause of the disorder is discovered.

Sometimes early onset strabismus is also named primary, in which case the eyes are healthy. Secondary strabismus is a consequence of an eye disease.

The strabismus terminology also includes consecutive forms, describing the cases that in time, spontaneously or as a consequence of extraocular muscle surgery, and changes the visual axes direction, from convergent to divergent or vice versa.

Primary importance of strabismus is that it can lead to amblyopia. The risk for it is much higher in unilateral forms—only one eye is constantly deviating. Consequently, due to asymmetric input, active suppression of the impulses from the deviating eye occurs, later leading to amblyopia. In alternating strabismus, the child switches fixation between the two eyes, and the risk of amblyopia is much lower. Nevertheless, in both forms, due to different visual axes direction, stereopsis is lost. Another possible consequence of strabismus is anomalous head posture. By turning or tilting the head, the patient seeks the position in which he or she still can maintain both eyes directed to the fixation point—this state is named orthotropia. Sometimes patients have manifest strabismus even in anomalous head position, but that position gives them better vision. The underlying cause can be nystagmus or the different tonus in antagonistic muscles.

2. Ophthalmologic examination of the child

2.1 Anamnesis

The ophthalmological examination begins with an anamnesis; when we talk about the examination of a child, it is actually about heteroanamnesis. The infor-mation is usually obtained from a parent or guardian of a child. There are general anamnesis (past illnesses), ophthalmic history, family history, drug taking, and drug allergy. Attention should be paid to premature birth, family history, and hereditary diseases in the family [4].

The general (hetero)anamnesis should also be very detailed. Important data are also about prenatal development—risk factors and possible complications in pregnancy. Intrauterine growth failure, the presence of other anomalies, or premature labor is associated with a higher frequency of strabismus. Even 35% of premature infants develop strabismus, often associated with higher refractive anomalies. Therefore, an ophthalmologic examination of each premature child is recommended, certainly within the first year of life, preferably at the age of 6 months.

Family anamnesis often reveals the existence of other family members who have strabism or refractive anomalies. If one parent squints, the risk of a child having strabism is 15%, and if both parents have strabismus, that risk is as high as 45%. If the family history is positive to strabismus, refractive errors, and weakness, an ophthalmic examination is required before the age of 3.

Ophthalmological anamnesis: It is important to find out when the strabismus occurred—in the first months of life or later, whether the occurrence is sudden, "overnight," or whether it was gradual, in the beginning only intermittent, becoming constant with time. It is important to know when the child is tired or sick and whether it changes during the day. Sometimes the eye is deviating only when the child is looking in the far distance or while "daydreaming" and at near fixation and with attention eyes that are straight. Some squints are manifest only under certain circumstances—for example, when exposed to the bright light (intermittent exotropia) or when the child wants to see some tiny details at near (accommodative esotropia). It is also important to know whether the strabismic angle is stable—increasing, decreasing, or constant through the follow-up. Sometimes parents are not sure about the direction of deviation. Photos or drawings of convergent and divergent forms of strabismus help parents to show what they see in their child. It is always necessary to ask whether the deviation changed the direction—sometimes early convergent strabismus with time changes to divergent type. Therefore the parents should be asked whether in the beginning there was an inward turn of the eye, toward the nose, only later to change to outward turn. Very important question is which eye is deviating—always the same or the child switches fixation between the eyes, while the other eye is deviating. Often the parents of the child with divergent squint say that they never know what the child is looking at. In vertical forms, parents usually say that in some gaze direction, child's eyes are looking strange or weird. Parents can also share the information about some unusual head position and whether that is present all the time awake or only when the child is trying to see something better. Sometimes the anomalous head position occurs only during prolonged looking in the same direction. The information about anomalous head position is also important in view of strabismus treatment prognosis. If there was a period in life when the patient constantly held the head in the same anomalous position, it might be presumed that it was for maintaining the learned binocularity that could return after surgical correction of strabismus. In sudden occurrence of strabismus, somewhat older child can tell it's parents that it sees double. Younger children are not able to tell that, but it can be noticed that the child squeezes one eye to avoid diplopia. The younger the child, the period of double vision will be shorter, because suppression will develop sooner, so sometimes parents forget about this information if not specifically asked.

2.2 Clinical examination

Inspection is the first part of the clinical examination of the patient with strabismus. Even when we talk to parents, we can observe the child—whether there is an impression of the wrong orientation of the sight axes and where the sight axes are oriented (convergent, divergent, and vertical strabismus) [5].

3. Evaluation of fixation and visual acuity

The visual function test methods depend on the age of the child.

By the age of 2 of the child, a subjective reflection may be used to examine the reflection of blinking on a very light pupil reflex, fixation, and the monitoring of the colorful objects that are offered to the child for looking at [6].

The first examination is binocular and then monocular: is the fixation of child's view on the object, is fixation maintained, and is the object of fixation followed. Fixation reflex can be examined at the 3–4 months of age.

Objective methods can cause optokinetic nystagmus (OKN), examine cortical visual evoked potentials (VEP), and evaluate visual acuity with a preferential looking test.

3.1 Determination of fixation type

Occlusion of one eye is made.

1. If the child instantly fixes the source of the light, whose reflex is in the center of the pupil, then it is central fixation.

2. If a child looks at the source of the light, but the eye which has to take the fixation does not come to the middle position, it is eccentric fixation.

3. If the baby does not fix with an eye, then there is no fixation at all.

4. Determination of visualization by test pictures (star and circle) that are projected on the retina.

3.2 Preferential looking test

The method of visual acuity that is based on the observation of the child's eyes, to which of the two offered fields will the child first look at (homogeneous gray and striped black and white). Children prefer to look at more interesting, striped objects. As the width of the black and white stripes becomes more and more like a gray homogeneous field, it is harder to spot the difference, and if the child is aware of the slightest difference between the stripes, the visual acuity is neat.

This method is suitable for using from the 4 months of age.

3.3 Examination of visual acuity in children 2: 4 years of age

After the child starts to speak, the visual acuity is examined by standardized tests with close-range and distance-based image optotypes. These are the first tests that examine the visual acuity quantitatively [7].

The most commonly used standardized tests are Lohnlein's tables and Lea symbols.

Lea test table consists of four symbols (circle, square, house, and heart) that are shown in each of the following order in a smaller size. Tested at 3 meters distance and not at 5 or 6 meters as well as other tests and less environment distracts the child. The same symbols can be used to examine visual acuity at close. The test is standardized according to Snellen's table.

3.4 Examination of visual acuity in children older than 4 years

The gold standard for testing is Snellen's tables. Snellen's board consists of rows of optotypes (letters, numbers, and hooks). Each part of Snellen's optotype corresponds to a visual angle of 1 minute, unlike the image optotypes that do not hold that rule, such as the smallest pictures of image optotypes that should match the visual acuity of 1.0, that actually correspond to the visual acuity of 0.66.

Landolt's rings are also based on the Snellen's principle (the width of the ring opening is 1 angular minute). The flaw is that it can only be used with the children who learned how to tell time.

3.5 Visual acuity test weaker than 0.1

It can be done with individual Snellen's optotypes. We approach the child gradually, and at the distance at which the optotype is properly recognized, we note the visual acuity in the form of a break. If a child from 1 meter of distance detects the direction of Snellen's largest optotype, then the visual acuity is 1/60. If the child does not reveal it, we ask him to count the fingers on our hand and write down where the child is at a distance (30 cm, right in front of the eye).

If we doubt the weaker eyesight, we are examining the sensation of light and the projection in the dark room. It is tested with a lamp at a distance of 1 meter and by turning on the light from the upper, lower, left, and right sides. We write down neat sense of light and projection as L+ P+.

4. Binocular vision tests/stereo vision tests

Binocular single vision is simultaneous viewing of both eyes at the same point of fixation, which realizes a single image of the object [8].

4.1 Binocular vision elements by worth

Simultaneous perception (at the same time, at the two corresponding retinal points of both eyes, a likeness of approximately the same size is created.)

Fusion reflex (a psycho-optical reflex that connects two figures to one if they are formed at corresponding points).

Stereovision (stereopsis—disparate characters merge with a sense of space and depth) or depth perception can be characterized as the highest degree of binocular vision.

4.2 Motor binocular vision component

Motility and ocular motor balance make the motor component of binocular vision. The muscular system of eye mobility has enabled the image of the fixation object to be held in the fovea in each eye individually, and that fusion segment is called the motor fusion.

Sensory component will at the level of the visual cortex of two visible impressions merge into one. The sensory component consists of a retinal correspondence and a reflection of binocular vision. Its basis is normal retinal correspondence thanks to which we see single using two eyes, because the characters formed centrally merge creating a single perception.

4.3 Tests for stereopsis examination

Testing with Bagolini's striated glasses is the most important test of simultaneous perception, because of its minimal dissociation results which are the most similar to the natural viewing of the patient [9]. The glass slides used in the test are longitudinally twisted and turn the small lamp into a luminous line vertical to the glass' striation. The straps are oriented right and left in front of the eye so that the lines are at right angles. The orientation of the line as the patient sees it is usually marked on the edge of the glass slide itself with dots. It is very important to know how the slides are oriented, because our interpretation of the test result depends on it. Usually they are set to have a right eye line at 135° and left at 45°. In the state of orthotropy and proper binocular vision, the patient sees two lines passing through the light itself, like the letter X. If there is strabismus and simultaneous perception, the patient will see both lines, but they will not cross in the light itself. If Bagolini's slides are oriented as indicated above (right line at 135°, left at 45°), the patient with esotropia sees two lines and one light on each one, and the lines will be crossed over the light (non-crossed double images). If it is a case of exotropy, the lines are crossed under the light (crossed double images). If there is a central scotoma on a stray eye, the line of the eye in the middle of the light will not be visible but only the ends of the line. Depending on their position, we can also find out whether they are associated with normal or anomalous retinal correspondence. Finally, in the case of suppressing a stray eye, the patient will see only one line—the one of the eye which is fixing the light.

This test can be performed not only in the straightforward but in different directions of view. It is advisable to examine the direction of view where the smallest, or visible, axis of the eye is the closest (e.g., in the V exotypically downward model) to assess whether a functional case with potential binocularity or only esthetic case (constant exclusion of one eye with Bagolini's). This test can also be performed after the prism adaptation test, whereby both sight axes are directed to the fixation object. Bagolini's striated glass is placed in front of the lenses, and the patient's responses are evaluated.

With the fusion test using the prisms, we can examine whether there is bifunctional fixation and what is the potential of motor and sensory fusion. In the test, we use a prism of strength of 14 or 15 diopters because the induced fusion motor displacement is large enough to be perceived. It is very good for small children within the first year of life; in older children the cooperation in this test is somewhat weaker.

The test is carried out by drawing the child's attention to the fixing object of fixation of the appropriate size and placing the base of the prism temporally.

Titmus test is tested with polarizing glasses. After the spectacles are placed, the respondents are given cards with different characters displayed in different depth positions. The first test is a test of the rough Fly-fly test. The person with stereo vision sees the fly in three dimensions, and the baby catches the wings of the fly with its fingers. The following is examined for the finer stereopsis: the characters are placed in rows, and in each row one character rises above the others. The last test is circle test, four circles within nine groups; one circle of each group rises. Titmus test quantifies the level of stereopsis in the angle seconds.

Lang test card is a screening test designed for early detection of problems with stereoscopic vision in children. Two versions of the test plates are available, which differ only according to the 3D objects to be recognized. The Lang test 1 displays a star, a cat, and a car, while the Land test 2 displays a moon, a truck, and an elephant, each of them appearing on a different level. No glasses are necessary for the Lang Stereo Test.

5. Hirschberg's test

Using the Hirschberg's test, we determine the size of the squinting angle depending on the position of the reflex position on the cornea when simultaneously illuminating both eyes.

The patient is said to look at the top of the lamp. The position of the light reflex in relation to the center of the cornea of one eye and the position of the reflex light of one in relation to the other eye are compared.

The difference in the position of reflection on the cornea of the right and left eye raises the suspicion of strabismus. If the reflex is shifted from the center of the eye nasally, the impression of divergent strabismus of that eye is obtained, if shifted temporally—convergent. Reflex shift upward points to hypotrophy and downward to hypertrophy of that eye. It is important to note that it is always necessary to compare the position of reflexes on the right and left eye, since sometimes it is seen that reflexes of both eyes are slightly decentralized. Only the difference in position indicates the existence of strabismus. In small children where measurement of the strabic angle is not yet possible by other methods, the deviation can be semiquantitatively determined by the reflex position. In this case 1 mm difference in the reflex position corresponds to the angle of about 7°. With this test we can easily examine the existence of angle difference in different directions of view. The child follows the source of light as we look at the change in the position of the reflex on the corneas.

The reflex shift for 1 mm is equal to the displacement of 7°, which is 15 DP.

According to the reflex position, the angle is determined according to the following anatomic determinations: if the reflex at the periphery of the pupil is 15° or 30 DP, the reflex in the center of the iris determines the angle of 30° or 60 PD; the limbus position determines the angle of 45° or 90PD.

Hirschberg test is fast and simple, but unfortunately not accurate enough. Both the specificity and the sensitivity are rather low.

There are cases of eccentric fixation where one could, based on corneal reflex position, presume the presence of strabismus that actually is not there (false positive, low specificity). Eccentric fixation is common in ectopia of macula lutea due to retinopathy of prematurity. Strabismus associated with eccentric fixation might be operated on only if the eccentric viewing eye is not the better, fixating eye. The angle formed by visual axis and central pupillary axis is called angle kappa, and it is present in most people. Positive angle kappa (nasal shift of the corneal reflex) gives the impression of divergent strabismus, whereas negative angle kappa (temporal shift of the corneal reflex) resembles convergent strabismus. The asymmetry of angle kappa between the eyes can arouse the suspicion of strabismus that actually is not present (false positive, low specificity). In small strabismic angles—microstrabismus—the difference in corneal light reflex position is too small to be detected (false negative, low sensitivity).

6. Brückner's test

A very fast, equally simple, but more sensitive test is a test of observation of red eye reflection of the bottom of the eye or the Brückner's test. It is easy to perform and is very accurate right in the first year of life; from about 4–5 months when foveal fixation is already developed, it has its value in small angles of squinting, anisometropia and amblyopia, high hypermometry and myopia, and cataracts in young, noncooperative children.

With simultaneous enlightenment of both eyes with ophthalmoscope light, through the ophthalmoscope, we see whether there are differences in intensity between the light of reflex of the right and left eye fundus. It is best to use a direct ophthalmoscope, where illumination and observation are coaxial. We sit on about 70 cm from the patient and several times briefly illuminate both eyes, to prevent narrowing of the pupils to the light.

Reflexes in the eye opening of the child facing the straight line will be dark, while the reflection of the eye in deflection will be significantly brighter.

The phenomenon arises because of the anatomical structure of the fovea itself, that is, the recesses, causing all the light that vertically falls on the fovea, that is, the foveola does not return to the ophthalmoscope but is reflected in the other direction in the eye of the patient—that is why the reflex of the eye fixed by the fovea is darker. With this test we can detect very small deviations of the position of the axes—but the deviation of 1–2° gives a difference in the light of the reflex. In addition to the detection of strabismus, this test also reveals the existence of refractive anomalies (amethropy and less anisometropia) by the analysis of light distribution in the pupil. Significant hypermetropia will be shown as inferiorly positioned bright semiprecious red reflection, while significant myopia will be shown as a super bright light half-moon in a red reflex.

The absence of a reflection from the eye bottom points to the blur of optical eye media (cornea, lens, or glass body). White or very bright reflexes (leukocytes) cause pathological changes in the eyelid, such as coloboma or retinoblastoma. It is important to note that even at this test, the accuracy of the detection of strabismus is not complete, because the difference in reflex can be caused by even greater anisometropies. From a highly amethropic eye, the beam of light is divergently reflected, so the reflex from such eye is dark, although the eye may be in deflection (falsely negative result).

7. Motility

When examining the eye movement, we first look at each eye separately (the other eye is folded by the hand) from the primary eye position in the direction of the action of each muscle in particular (movements of duction). The movements of one eye are called duction. The upward movement is elevation or supraduction and downward depression or infraduction. The inward move, toward the nose, is adduction and outward abduction. Torsional or rotational movements can be examined by head tilt—head tilt to the shoulder on the same side as the eye under investigation will cause incycloduction and to the opposite shoulder excycloduction. The movements of both eyes in the same direction are called versions. Right gaze is called dextroversion and left levoversion, upgaze supraversion, and downgaze infraversion. Oblique gaze directions are called supra-dextro/−levoversion and infra-dextro/−levoversion. Torsional movements can be examined here as well—right head tilt will cause levocycloversion (rotation to the left) and left head tilt dextrocycloversion (rotation to the right) [10].

The movements of both eyes in the opposite direction are called vergencies. If the eyes simultaneously move toward the nose, it is called convergence and outward—divergence. Simultaneous incyclorotation of both eyes usually accompanies convergence—this is called incyclovergence and with excyclorotation with divergence, excyclovergence.

Due to relative position of the extraocular muscles and eye globe, isolated action of vertical muscles—superior and inferior rectus muscles—should be examined in slight abduction (cca 20–25°) and superior and inferior oblique muscles in more accentuated adduction (cca 50°), because in the middle there is a combination of rectus and oblique muscle actions in the sense of elevation and depression.

The primary eye position exists when eyes fix an object that is at their height straight in front of them or in infinity (beyond 6 meters). All other positions in the eye that come up with the action of certain muscles are the diagnostic (secondary) positions of the eyes that are in the direction of the action.

There are nine viewpoints—the primary (straightforward), the central vertical position (straight and up, straight and down), and cardinal (up and left, left, down and left, up and right, right, down and right).

When there is a case of very young children, who still have no developed attention, eye movements are tested with a doll's head maneuver. Turning the head to one side causes a reflex eye shift to the opposite side, unless there is a mechanical restriction of movement or a myogenic weakness.

8. Cover/uncover test

The most accurate test for the detection of manifest strabismus is the eye cover test or the cover test [11].

The patient fixes the object in front of him. Penlight could be used for fixation, but it is better to use a target with shape (picture or an optotype), especially at near, because it stimulates accommodation, and the influence of accommodation on the deviation could be assessed in the same time.

The examiner alternately covers and uncovers only one eye. Coverage and uncoverage are performed several times, and we analyze eye positioning movements.

Cover test–test of coverage, the occluder covers the fixing eye. It follows the action of the other, uncovered eye.

Uncover test—detection test, the occluder uncovers-detects the fixing eye. When detecting, we follow the movement setting of the recently uncovered eye.

In the orthophoria, the eyes are not moving, no adjustment movement is present, and the cover test is negative.

Cover test is always tested with and without correction and in different directions of looking.

The test is very sensitive—it can reveal deviations as small as 1°. There are motoric and sensoric prerequisites that have to be fulfilled to make the test meaningful and valid—patient's fovea must be healthy, the eye must not be blind, and the eye must be able to move to take up fixation.

If the deviating eye is deeply amblyopic, it is hard for the patient to take up the fixation. Such eye often makes wondering movements trying to fixate the object, and sometimes it is hard to detect the direction of the first movement. In patients with nystagmus, it is also hard to detect the direction of the uncovered eye. Another disadvantage of the test is that it is not suitable and reliable in very small children (first year of life).

Cover test is followed by alternating cover test that can reveal latent strabismus (heterophoria) or additional latent component of manifest strabismus. The cover is alternated between the eyes and relatively fast, so the patient is fixating only monocularly—either by the right or the left eye. To relax the fusional mechanisms, the cover is held in front of the eye a little bit longer. The eye under cover could be observed from the side to see the slow slide of the eye into the anomalous position of muscular tone balance. When it stops, we quickly shift the cover on the other eye and observe now uncovered eye—what kind of movement and in what direction it makes. The magnitude of latent deviation indicates the amount of necessary effort to keep orthotropia—if the latent deviation is large, the demand on the central nervous system for keeping binocularity is substantial and can cause asthenopic symptoms. The direction of movement, just like in cover test, tells us what kind of heterophoria is present. In esophoria the eye shift is outward and in exophoria in the opposite direction—inward. In vertical phorias, if the right eye comes from above, and the left from below, we designate the movement as right over left (R/L) or plus vertical difference (+VD). If the movement is in the opposite direction—the left eye comes from above and the right from below—it is left over right deviation (L/R) or minus vertical difference (−VD).

Alternating cover test is followed by uncover test. After a few seconds of occlusion of one eye, the eye is uncovered and observed to see is there a fusional movement in order to regain binocularity. This test is very important because it give us information about the capacity of central fusional mechanisms that maintain binocularity. If the stress of dissociation under cover is too much for the system, the uncovered eye will stay in deviated position. Sometimes at near the fusional movement regains orthotropia, and at distance testing the uncovered eye does not move and stays in tropia. This is often the case in intermittent exotropia. Sometimes the uncovered eye does not reach the position of orthotropia; the deviation is decreased only for its latent component to the level of manifest deviation. If that manifest strabismic angle is small enough, visual system can even in this position preserve some level of binocularity, albeit anomalous. Uncover test can also be utilized in another important aspect. It can qualitatively determine the strength of eye dominance in patients with strabismus. The straight-looking eye is covered in order to shift the fixation to the strabismic eye. After a few seconds of stabilizing fixation on the accommodative object, the cover is removed. The speed of fixation shift to the uncovered eye indicates the strength of dominance but also the presence and level of amblyopia of the strabismic eye [12]. This could be semi-quantified, according to the length of holding fixation by the uncovered eye in bi-ocular viewing conditions. Based on this quantification, the length of dominant eye occlusion for treating amblyopia can be recommended even in preverbal children.

9. Strabismic angle measurement

There are objective and subjective methods for strabismic angle measurement. Objective methods include prism cover test (PCT) and Hirschberg test. The latter has already been described, together with its drawbacks, but usually it is the first test used for orientation about the direction and magnitude of deviation to shorten the measurement with PCT. Subjective methods are based on patient's response and therefore are suitable for older children and adults. They include Maddox cross method, Hess-Lancaster test, and tangent screen. They are based on diplopia recognition, and the dissociation is elicited by colored (red/green) or stripped glasses (Maddox rod) through which the patient looks. Dissociation could be also by physical separation of images, like in classic Maddox wing that is used for near deviation measurement or in major haploscope (synoptophore) with separate projection of images in the right and the left eye. In Hess-Lancaster or tangent screen method, the deviation is measured on calibrated screen in front of the patient on which the colored lights are projected. In Maddox cross method, calibrated cross with numbers representing degrees of deviation related to the distance on which the patient is seated and point light in the center is used for measurement. The dissociation is elicited by dark red glass in front of one eye, while the patient fixates the light in the center of the cross with the other eye. The patient is asked if he/she sees one or both lights—red and white. If the patient sees only one light, either orthophoria is present (both visual axes are directed toward the light) or there is suppression of one eye. If there are two lights—red and white—heterophoria is present. According to the relative position of the red and white light, the direction of deviation of the eye with the red glass is determined. If the red glass is in front of the right eye (the patient fixates the white light with the left eye), and the red light is on the right side of the white light, there is uncrossed diplopia, indicating esophoria. If the red light is on the left side of the white, crossed diplopia is present indicating exophoria. Similar is with vertical deviations—red over white light speaks for hypophoria of the eye with the red glass and red below white for hyperphoria of the same eye. The position of the red light on the Maddox cross determine strabismic angle in degrees.

The most accurate method for strabismic angle measurement is prism cover test (PCT). Similar to cover test, there are subtypes of this test—one that measures manifest deviation called simultaneous prism cover test (SPCT) and the one measuring the whole deviation (manifest and latent) called alternating prism cover test (APCT). This enables the determination of heterophoria component in the whole strabismic angle.

In SPCT, the prism with apex directed toward the direction of deviation is placed in front of the strabismic eye simultaneously with placing the occluder in front of the straight-looking eye. We observe the residual eye movement and change the prism strength as long as the eye under prism does not move anymore. This is the way to measure the manifest part of strabismic angle.

SPCT is followed by APCT in which we leave the found strength of prism in front of the eye, but now we shift the occluder between the eyes and observe possible movements. If there is a residual movement, we increase the strength of the prism to the point when eyes are still. The found prism strength equals the whole strabismic angle—added manifest and latent deviation. It is important to know that sometimes in measuring esotropia with very weak or no binocular potential, it is impossible to achieve the state without eyes' movements—there is always the same small outward movement from eso position. One should decrease the strength of the prism to the value when the movement increases and again increase the strength to the point of smallest outward movement—state of small microstrabismus—and this is the true value of measured angle.

Both tests are performed at near and far distance fixations, but in small children sometimes this is not possible. Some entertaining distance fixation objects (animated feature or dancing mechanical toy giving attractive sounds) significantly improve child's cooperation.

10. Skiascopy/retinoscopy

The retinoscope is an instrument used to objectively determine the refractive strength of the eye. It works on the principle that the retinoscopic probe projects a beam of light into the eye and then observes the light reflecting on the retina. Depending on the refractive strength of the eye, the beam of the light coming out of the eye will be of different character, with the myopia of the radiating ray converging, at the hypermetropia the output rays diverge, and in the emetropy the radiating rays leaving the eye are parallel.

During examination, the examiner performs small movements with the retinoscope up/down and left/right, and in the pupil observes the movement of the "shadow of light," and then uses different lenses in the eye to neutralize the reflex.

In the miope, the light reflex moves in the opposite direction to the retinoscope movement, and in the hypermetropic light, reflexion moves in the same direction.

Skiascopy is performed only when cycloplegic accommodations are pharmacologically excluded. To achieve cycloplegia in newborns and infants, tropicamide in 0.5% concentration is used. In older children 1% tropicamide is used. The drops should be instilled twice, 10 minutes apart, and the maximal cycloplegia is reached in 35–40 minutes. In this age, 1% cyclopentolate, minimally stronger acting cycloplegic, could also be used. Maximal cycloplegia is reached in 40–50 minutes. Atropine in 1% concentration is due to prolonged cycloplegia rarely used, but sometimes in children with limited cooperation or if variable result of refraction is found with shorter acting medications, this cycloplegic could also be used. The skiascopy is useful in prescribing corrective lenses to patients who cannot undergo subjective examination of visual acuity (adults with limited intellectual ability and children with a high accommodative eye power that must be excluded because it can mask an objective refraction error).

11. Fundoscopy

In children with strabismus, inspection of the eye fundus is unavoidable part of the examination. Organic disease as the cause of the eye deviation must be excluded. Posterior pole scars, coloboma, but also malignancies such as retinoblastoma can lead to instability or loss of fixation and strabismus. Unfortunately, peripherally situated tumors do not have to give signs of the disease in the beginning. Therefore, ophthalmoscopy in mydriasis is recommended even within usual, routine ophthalmological examination in children. Indirect binocular ophthalmoscope is the instrument of choice, due to its simplicity, speed, and the possibility to examine peripheral parts of the retina. It is recommended to use the least light intensity that still gives reliable picture to encourage child's cooperation. The attention and gaze direction change could be achieved by sound toys, like in motility exam, in order to get a glimpse on peripheral retina. Loupe of 20 diopter is usually used, as it gives optimal relation between field of vision and image magnification. If some pathological change is found, other loupes with less dioptric power (e.g., 16 d), giving bigger image, can be used, but the field of vision is less here. They are also suitable for posterior pole examination.

Author details

Suzana Konjevoda[1], Neda Striber[2*], Samir Čanović[1] and Ana Didović Pavičić[1]

1 General Hospital Zadar, Zadar, Croatia

2 Childrens' Hospital Zagreb, Zagreb, Croatia

*Address all correspondence to: striber.neda@gmail.com

IntechOpen

References

[1] Willshaw H, Scotcher S, Beaty S. In: Willshaw HE, editor. A Handbook of Paediatric Ophthalmology. Birmingham, UK; 2000

[2] Čelić M, Dorn V. Strabizam i Nistagmus. Zagreb: Medicinska Naklada; 2004

[3] Jin YH. Strabismus. Ulsan: UUP; 2001. pp. 205-225

[4] Lang J. Strabismus: Diagnostik, Schielformen, Therapie. 4. izdanje ed. Bern, Gottingen, Toronto, Seattle: Hans Huber Verlag; 1994

[5] Rosenbaum AL, Santiago AP, editors. Clinical Strabismus Management. Philadelphia, London, Toronto, Montreal, Sydney, Tokyo: W.B. Saunders Company; 1999

[6] Bremond-Gignac D, Copin H, Lapillonne A, Milazzo S, European Network of Study and Research in Eye Development. Visual development in infants: Physiological and pathological mechanisms. Current Opinion in Ophthalmology. 2011;22(Suppl):S1-S8

[7] Dorn LJ. Vid i vidna oštrina u male djece. Paediatria Croatica. 2004;48(Suppl 1):247-254

[8] Von Noorden GK. Binocular Vision and Ocular Motility. St Louis: Mosby; 1996

[9] Petrinović DJ. The Script from Continuing Education Course: "Diagnostic and Therapeutic Procedures in Strabology and Pediatric Ophthalmology". Zadar; 2008-2017

[10] Boergen KP. Oblique Muscles Disorders. Courses of Continuing Education: "Diagnostic and Therapeutic Procedures in Strabology and Pediatric Ophthalmology". Zadar; 2008-2017

[11] Von Noorden GK, Campos EC. Binocular Vision and Ocular Motility: Theory and Management of Strabismus. 6th ed. St. Louis, Missouri: Mosby; 2002

[12] Dickey CF, Metz HS, Stewart SA, Scott WE. The diagnosis of amblyopia in cross-fixation. Journal of Pediatric Ophthalmology and Strabismus. 1991;28(3):171-175

Section 3

Disorders of the Eye Motility System

Chapter 4

Nystagmus

Ivana Mravicic, Selma Lukacevic, Maja Bohac,
Maja Pauk-Gulic and Vlade Glavota

Abstract

Nystagmus is an involuntary rhythmical movement of the eyes. The cause of
nystagmus is a disruption in the afferent, central or efferent parts of the eye
movement system. If it happens in the first few months of life during the sensitive
period of visual development, it is most often a case of infantile nystagmus. On the
other hand, the majority of nystagmus in adult age is caused by some neurological
disorder, and it is usually called acquired nystagmus. The important role of an
ophthalmologist is to recognize the origin of nystagmus. Acquired forms are usually
caused by some neurological disorders and do not belong in our field of treatment.
However, most of the nystagmus types in a child's age require ophthalmological
treatment. When we have a child with nystagmus, we have to enable the development of the visual system and help fixation and fovealization by the dampening of
nystagmus. If the reason of nystagmus is of ocular origin, we have to treat the
underlying disease. Optical treatment by glasses, contact lenses or magnifying
devices is usually reasonable. In some cases when the patient has abnormal head
posture, it is possible to treat nystagmus by surgery. Some medications are used in
several types of nystagmus as well as some new developing treatments.

Keywords: nystagmus, infantile nystagmus, acquired nystagmus, spasmus nutans,
albinismus, artificial divergence, Anderson surgery, Kestenbaum surgery

1. Introduction

When examining the patients with nystagmus, we should start with the medical
history. One of the most important questions, especially in a child's age, is at what
age nystagmus started (infantile, benign form starts no later than 3 months of age).
Nystagmus usually consists of slow pursuit movement or drift which is followed by
a fast (jerk) or slow (pendular) movement of refixation. Though the first slow
movement is pathological, nystagmus is usually named after the second, fast
refixation movement. When the second movement is fast, nystagmus is called
"jerk", and in the cases when second movement is slow, nystagmus is called "pendular". When describing nystagmus we usually describe the direction of the movement that can be horizontal, vertical, rotatory or chaotic as well as the magnitude of
amplitude and frequency. It is important to emphasize that in cases when the
movements of both eyes are asymmetric, meaning that eyes do not have the same
amplitude, frequency or direction (dissociated nystagmus) or eyes moving in
opposite directions (disconjugate nystagmus), we have to consider that as an
alarming sign of central cause of nystagmus and send the patient immediately to a
neurologist. Besides doing the clinical analysis of nystagmus, we can record eye

movements by electrooculography. By using eye movement recording tests, we can analyze eye movements in detail and help better analysis of nystagmus in clinical research.

As ophthalmologists we have to pay special attention to eye conditions that are accompanied or caused by nystagmus. During a complete ophthalmological clinical examination of the eyes in the children with nystagmus, it is important to pay attention to the preferred head posture and associated eye abnormalities and take care that monocular visual acuity can be different if one eye is closed, so it is wise when performing visual acuity tests to dampen instead of close the non-tested eye [1, 2].

2. Types of nystagmus

Nystagmus is a complicated disease that most of us do not see every day in our offices.

According to its origin, nystagmus is usually divided in physiological, infantile and acquired [3]. An ophthalmologist has an important role to recognize the origin of nystagmus. Acquired nystagmus is usually caused by some neurological causes, and this complex disorder is in the field of neurologists as well as ear, nose and throat (ENT) specialists and not in our field of treatment. However, we should recognize the type of nystagmus and help localize the disruption. As ophthalmologists, we usually treat nystagmus in childhood. Most of the nystagmus types in a child's age are benign, and they do not require additional neurological workup [4, 5].

After medical history and clinical examination in the child with nystagmus, we can perform measurements of nystagmus by electronystagmography, as well as measurements of the afferent part of the system with visually evoked potential (VEP), optical coherence tomography (OCT) or electro-retinogram tests.

2.1 Physiological nystagmus

Since the visual acuity is degraded by image slip across the retina more than 2–3°/s, some nystagmus-like movements of the eyes are physiological and unconsciously used in everyday activity (**Table 1**).

Physiological fixational nystagmus	Nystagmus-like movements
Optokinetic	Microsaccade
Gaze evoked	Microtremor
Caloric	Slow drift
Rotatory	

Table 1.
Physiological fixational nystagmus and nystagmus-like movements.

There are several systems that are connecting the eyes (afferent part), structures in the brain and eye movement system (efferent part). Each of them is responsible and important in the cases when our body is moving or rotating or when we are fixing a moving target (**Table 2**) [3].

	Afferent visual system	Vestibular system		Neural integrator
Function	Provides image to guide eye movements	Moves eyes in response to self-motion		Maintain eccentric gaze in the presence of moving target
Anatomy	Retina Optic nerve Optic chiasm	Central	Peripheral	Medial vestibular nucleus Nucleus prepositus hypoglossus Flocculus Interstitial nucleus of Cajal

Table 2.
Eye movement systems.

2.2 Nystagmus in childhood

Benign nystagmus in childhood can be divided in several forms:

Idiopathic infantile nystagmus

Ocular/sensory nystagmus

Latent (manifest/latent) nystagmus

Spasmus nutans

Typical features of each form are listed in **Table 3**.

Type of nystagmus	Infantile nystagmus syndrome	Sensoric nystagmus	Manifest/latent nystagmus	Spasmus nutans
Onset of nystagmus	3–4 months	3–4 months	3–4 months	6 months–2 years
Additional eye findings	Early esotropia syndrome	Congenital cataract Cloudy cornea Albinism Congenital macular disease Optic nerve hypoplasia	Early esotropia syndrome	Head nodding
Visual acuity	Variable	Poor	Variable	Good
Prognosis	Recedes by the age of 8–9 years	No change	No change	Recedes in 1–2 years
Treatment	Visual aids, prisms, surgery	Treatment of underlying disease, visual aids	Visual aids, surgery	None

Table 3.
Benign nystagmus of childhood.

2.2.1 Idiopathic infantile nystagmus

Idiopathic infantile nystagmus is a primary motor dysfunction of unknown origin with no ocular pathology present. In some cases, it can be connected to some genotype but without a clear phenotypic pattern [6, 7]. Inherited forms are usually X-linked form in the FERM domain on Xq26.2 chromosome [8] or autosomal dominant situated at the chromosome 6p12 (NYS2) [9], 7p11 (BYS3) or 13q (NYS4) [10].

Idiopathic infantile nystagmus is probably present from birth but typically becomes noticeable in the first several months of life when a child starts to fixate. If it develops later, we have to suspect other kinds of nystagmus. It starts as a pendular form, later transforms into the jerk type and usually recedes spontaneously up to the 9th year of life, although it is usually present for lifetime. Idiopathic infantile nystagmus is usually horizontal and symmetrical but can have a rotatory component as well. Although it is typical that patients with infantile nystagmus do not have oscillopsia, they sometimes have head shaking or nodding, and it is also typical that nystagmus disappears during sleep. Some recent studies of patients with infantile nystagmus showed downregulation of the visual cortex which is responsible for motion processing (MT/V5 area) [11]. Typically patient with this kind of nystagmus does not have optokinetic nystagmus, and vestibulo-ocular reflex is disrupted [12]. Infantile nystagmus often (even up to 50%) comes with esotropia and is combined with some vertical movement disorders (congenital form of fourth muscle palsy or dissociated vertical deviation). Such a combination is then called infantile esotropia syndrome.

Infantile nystagmus is typically increasing when attempting to fixate a small visual object. The majority of children can dampen eye movements in convergence or some other eccentric direction of gaze. In the preferred position, sometimes called "null or neutral zone", nystagmus is dampening, so the fixation and fovealization are better, and children often have compensatory head position [13, 14]. In patients with infantile nystagmus, the development of the visual acuity is variable. Visual acuity can be 20/20 but sometimes it can be severely reduced.

2.2.2 Ocular/sensory nystagmus

This is a kind of nystagmus which develops in cases when, during the early visual development (the first few months of life), the development of vision is not possible because of anatomical changes or organic defects in the eye. Disorders of the eye can be obvious, but sometimes they are subtle and not easy to define [15]. The cause of sensory nystagmus is inadequate image formation in fovea which results in disruption between afferent and efferent system and causes disturbances of oculomotor control. The most common causes are diseases of the eye such as congenital cataract, albinism, corneal opacities as well as developmental abnormalities of the optic disc and retina such as Leber's amaurosis, achromatopsia or stationary night blindness [16]. Specific form of sensory strabismus is uniocular nystagmus in deep amblyopia (Heimann-Bielschowsky phenomenon).

2.2.2.1 Congenital cataract

Congenital cataract is opacification of the lens present at birth and may be responsible for amblyopia, sensory nystagmus and strabismus. The incidence varies between 2 and 4 in 10,000 worldwide [17].

The vast majority of congenital cataracts are bilateral, roughly between 60 and 70%. Identifiable cause of the cataract can be found in only half of them. Unilateral cataracts are mainly sporadic, found in otherwise healthy infants [17]. When they are associated with other local or system abnormalities, unilateral cataracts are usually found in eyes with other ocular abnormalities, and bilateral cataracts are mainly associated with system disorders (**Table 4**).

Not every lens opacification is equally important for normal vision development. The most sight threatening is if opacifications are central, more than 3 mm, located from central to the posterior parts of the lens. While sensory nystagmus usually develops in bilateral congenital cataracts, strabismus may occur in unilateral and bilateral cataracts.

Cataract	Unilateral	Bilateral		
Associated abnormality	Persistent foetal vasculature Posterior lenticonus/lentiglobus Anterior segment abnormalities Chorioretinal coloboma	Genetic malformations	Genetic mutations	*AD* *AR* *X-linked*
			Chromosomal abnormalities	*21 trisomy* *18 trisomy* *5p partial deletion*
		Metabolic disorders	*Galactosemia* *Wilson's disease* *Hypocalcemia* *DM*	
		Intrauterine infections	*Rubella*, Rubeola* *HSV, CMV, HZV, EBV* *Toxoplasmosis* *Syphilis*	

*Rubella is the most common intrauterine infection causing congenital cataract; DM, diabetes mellitus; HSV, herpes simplex virus; CMV, Cytomegalovirus; HZV, herpes zoster virus; EBV, Epstein–Barr virus.

Table 4.
Associated abnormalities in unilateral and bilateral cataracts.

Nystagmus is found in at least 24% of eyes with bilateral cataract, being thought to be a poor predicting factor for developing normal visual acuity [18].

As the risk of amblyopia is the greatest in the earliest months of life, it is of crucial importance to detect the cataract as soon as possible. That is why all infants must be screened for congenital cataracts immediately after birth and from 6 to 8 weeks of life. Screening is based on examination of red reflex. Any shadow in the reflex, absence or whitening of the reflex is an indication for complete ophthalmology examination [19]. On ophthalmology exam, it is essential to have a clear picture of fundus which is not blurred by opacification of the lens [17]. The more obscured fundus means that the vision development is more affected, and that determines timing of the surgery.

In cooperation with a pediatrician, set of laboratory examinations should be performed, even in cases without the presence of notable system abnormalities. If dysmorphic features are present, a genetic test should be suggested. Laboratory tests that should be done are TORCH titers; venereal disease research laboratory test (VDRL test); serum levels of calcium, phosphorus and blood glucose; and urine analysis for reducing substances (raised in galactosemia), galactokinase (raised in Fabry's disease), amino acids (raised in Lowe syndrome), calcium and phosphorus [19].

2.2.2.2 Albinism

Albinism is a disorder which is characterized by reduced pigmentation of the skin, hair and eyes caused by inborn defects in melanin biogenesis and distribution. The defect can be present as an isolated form or, less frequently, as a part of the syn-dromes (Chediak-Higashi, Hermansky-Pudlak, Waardenburg) [20]. Although four genes are known to cause autosomal recessive form, it seems that, only in one-third of the patients with albinism, mutations in known genes are confirmed [21]. If the lack of pigmentation is present in the skin, hair and eyes, the disorder is called oculocutaneous albinism (OCA); if the hypopigmentation is present only in the eyes, it is called ocular albinism (OA) [22]. Pigments have multiple functions in the development and protection of the visual system. Although the exact molecular mechanisms are not yet completely understood, it is well known that pigment is crucial in some critical steps of the visual development as well as a factor of protection of damaging light and cellular protection by being a trap for free radicals [23]. Important features of ocular albinism that causes reduced visual acuity are macular hypoplasia and abnormal decussation of the visual pathways [24, 25]. Because of the reduced visual acuity in patients with albinism amblyopia, nystagmus and strabismus often develop. Macular hypoplasia is the most important factor responsible for the reduced visual acuity in patients with albinism and is easily diagnosed by inspection (lack of foveal pit, abnormal growth of blood vessels) and confirmed by OCT (optical coherence tomography). Another important feature is the abnormal decussation of the visual pathways. In a normal eye, one half of the nerve fibers decussate to the contralateral side. On the other side, in patients with albinism, 75–85% of fibers project to the contralateral side [26]. The reason for that is lack of melanin in the specific time of development when melanin and its precursors have an important role in linking reception in the retina and perception in the brain [27].

With the clinical picture of the nystagmus alone, it is not possible to tell the difference between this kind of nystagmus and idiopathic infantile type. However, in this type visual acuity is severely reduced with no chances of improvement in contrast to the idiopathic form where the visual acuity can be normal. This type of nystagmus does not reduce during the years.

2.2.3 Latent nystagmus

Latent/manifest nystagmus is benign, jerk kind of nystagmus that starts early in the childhood. Although this type of nystagmus is bilateral and conjugated, the main characteristic is that the nystagmus is not visible (or much less visible) when both eyes are open. It increases when one eye is closed. Other typical feature of latent nystagmus is that it changes direction. The fast phases are always towards the open eye. When the right eye is closed, it beats left, and when the left eye is closed, fast phase is right [28]. Sometimes this kind of nystagmus is called fusion defect nystagmus (FDN) because it is present (or more pronounced) with one eye closed when fusion is disrupted [29]. This kind of nystagmus is usually combined with other anatomical eye abnormalities, and most often it is part of the early esotropia syndrome [30].

2.2.4 Spasmus nutans

Spasmus nutans is a benign nystagmus of childhood which is dissociated (different amplitudes, directions or frequencies between two eyes). The frequency is usually high, movement pendular, with a small amplitude, and disconjugated oscillations. The movements can be horizontal, vertical or torsional. It typically starts later than the idiopathic form, usually at the age of 4–12 months. If it starts after 3 years of age, the possibility of an intracranial tumor is strong. It is often preceded by the head nodding several months before the appearance of the nystagmus itself. Spasmus nutans is a specific form that can be a problem for diagnostics since there is no certain clinical sign that can differentiate this kind of nystagmus from the nystagmus caused by neurological problems (tumors in diencephalon) [31]. It is necessary for this kind of nystagmus to perform a complete neurological and endocrinological workup. Spasmus nutans typically disappears spontaneously in the 4th year of life [31].

2.3 Acquired nystagmus

As mentioned in (**Table 2**), several systems working in synchrony are responsible for involuntary movements of our eyes. The disorder that creates

Affected system	Afferent visual system	Vestibular system	Neural integrator
Etiology	Neuroblastoma	Tumors (brainstem)	Cerebellar diseases
	Optic nerve glioma	Stroke (brainstem)	Brainstem diseases
		Degenerative diseases	Drugs
		Drugs	

Table 5.
Acquired nystagmus.

pathological nystagmus can be situated in some parts of these systems or in the surrounding parts of the brain, brain stem and cerebellum. Most often the reasons are strokes or mass lesions, trauma, multiple sclerosis, some malformations and drugs (**Table 5**).

Another important characteristic that usually makes difference between acquired and benign forms is that acquired nystagmus is usually combined with other neurological signs like nausea, vomiting, headache, vertigo or tinnitus. In some cases the type or direction of the nystagmus can help us localize the place of lesion. For example, vestibular system is responsible for moving eyes in the opposite direction of the moving of the head. Both sides of system work in balance. When one side of the system is damaged, balance is lost, and the eyes will beat towards the not affected side and do not change side when the gaze changes direction. It is typical for this kind of disruption that nystagmus is increasing when the patient is not fixing. Lesions of the peripheral part of vestibular system (labyrinth) are accompanied by ataxia, vertigo and other signs of disturbances of the vegetative system. On the other hand, in the cases when damage is in the brainstem, often involving vestibular nuclei (fasciculus longitudinalis medialis), the direction of nystagmus is changing with the direction of the gaze, with the amplitude increasing when looking at the affected side. The intensity of nystagmus is increasing with fixation. In the cases of cerebellum diseases, nystagmus is increasing with fixation, more pronounced with the bigger amplitude and slower frequency when the gaze is towards the affected side. Vertical nystagmus is usually of central origin, and in some cases, it can be caused by excessive sedative medications intake. Acquired nystagmus can be a life-threatening condition which sometimes requires urgent neurological treatment [3]. Although in child's age the incidence of acquired nystagmus is smaller than in adult groups (17% in children compared to 40% in adult groups) [4, 5]. In our clinical work, it is of crucial importance when examining a child with nystagmus to notice the signs that are warning us that nystagmus is neurological in its origin, which means that the cause which is central does not require our treatment but needs neurological examinations, imaging and treatment [1].

Signs for neurological cause of nystagmus are:

• Neurological symptoms (vertigo, nausea, headache, vomiting)

• Existence of the additional signs on the eyes (oedema of optic nerve, RAPD)

• Nystagmus which is disconjugated or dissociated

• Oscillopsia

• Existence of optokinetic reflex

• Appearance of nystagmus after the 4th months of age [1]

3. Treatment

In the cases when nystagmus is acquired, it is necessary to treat the reason that caused nystagmus. That treatment is usually in the hands of neurologists or neuro-surgeons. When we have a child with some type of benign nystagmus, the primary goal is to improve proper development of the visual system which is in the hands of ophthalmologists. When the baby is born, the visual system is not fully developed, and it needs proper stimulation at the proper time for the cells in visual parts of the brain to develop to their full potential. We can say that a child has to learn how to see. Children with nystagmus often have refractive errors such as astigmatisms, myopia or hyperopia, given prescription can enable better development of the visual system and with improvement of fixation and fovealization nystagmus can dampen. In the cases of very poor visual acuity, some magnifying visual aids can be helpful [32].

Often children with nystagmus can have abnormal head positon to enable better fixation so the optical axis of the glasses is not the same as the visual axis of the eye. In cases like that it is wise to prescribe contact lenses. The reason of the preferred position of the head is so called null zone of nystagmus. Certain types of nystagmus have eye position in which nystagmus is less pronounced. By abnormal head posi-tion, the child is positioning the eyes in the preferred position where nystagmus is dampening. Prescribing the prismatic correction (base towards the head turn) can shift the null zone and correct head position. Prism correction can correct only mild head turn and the does not have permanent effect so cannot be prescribed like a definite therapy. Bigger amounts of prism correction are heavy and cause chromatic aberration, and Fresnel prisms will degrade visual acuity.

In the cases when the preferred position is bigger than 10°, there is a possibility to perform surgery on the eye muscles to move the eyes in the direction of the head turn, in order to shift the dampening zone from the decentralized position to straight ahead, to enable the patient a better and easier fixation. When considering a possibility of surgery, we have to think that some kinds of nystagmus spontaneously dampen by the age of 8–9 years, so the surgery can be planned in older children.

Most commonly performed surgeries are:

Anderson type of surgery

Kestenbaum type of surgery

Artificial convergence

Y-splitting

Posterior suture (Faden surgery)

Anderson type of surgery consists of recession of horizontal muscles of both eyes. Which muscles will be operated depends on the position of the eye and the head. Anderson started with the recession of one muscle on each eye with the idea that with the recession of the muscle he will weaken the tension and contact between the eye and the muscle which can help in the dampening of the nystagmus [33]. But the main effect of this kind of surgery is shifting the gaze direction in to the dampening zone. His original idea was recession of yoke muscles of 4 mm [33]. After his idea many modifications are made from other authors with different amounts of recession but taking into consideration that the amount must be symmetrical on both eyes in order to prevent induction of strabismus. The advantage of this method is that we are not only shifting eyes in the right direction but weakening the contact between the eye and the muscle and by that helping to dampen nystagmus.

In some cases, it is impossible to correct the head positioning only with recessions, so we have to add resections. That kind of surgery is named after Kestenbaum who published his method at the same year as Anderson [34]. Depending on the position of the head, a combination of recessions and resections is performed. This kind of surgery can be done on vertical and oblique muscles in cases when the patient is lifting, lowering or tilting the head [35]. During the years, many modifications of these surgeries have been done, mostly with recommendations for bigger amounts of surgery. Originally, Kestenbaum proposed recessions and resections of 5 mm; one of the most popular recommendations is done by Parks "5,6,7,8 procedure" with 13 mm of surgery in each eye [36]. Calhoun, Harley, Nelson and Pratt-Johnson suggested "augmented Parks surgery"; some of them prefer up to 10 mm of recess resect surgery [37, 38].

A different type of surgery is recommended for patients who are turning the head when looking at far distance and having their head straight when reading. The reason for dampening of nystagmus is convergence that they are using for near work. In such patients, we can perform a procedure called "artificial divergence", meaning that we create a latent divergence by surgery so the patient has to use convergence when looking at far distance (like during reading at near) and by that is dampening the nystagmus. When performing this type of surgery, we have to be sure that the patient has binocularity (possibility to use both eyes together); otherwise we will not achieve the goal of the surgery. It is always wise to simulate the wanted postoperative position by using prisms before the surgery. In the case of artificial divergence, we can check the amount of wanted divergence by putting prisms on both eyes and checking whether the patient is converging or accommodating and by that better estimate the amount of the needed surgery [39].

Some patients are changing their preferred head position, sometimes turning left and other time right with dampening nystagmus when the eyes are in convergent position. Often they do not have binocularity as the group mentioned previously, so we cannot use their active convergence to dampen nystagmus. In cases like this, Y-splitting of the medial rectus can be performed. By splitting both medial recti in two half up to 15 mm from the insertions, we create two arms of one muscle and fixate them away from each other. The exact position of placing the respective arms is calculated using a mathematical model in which axial length and angle of additional squinting must be added to the formula. By this kind of surgery, we block action of medial muscle only in adduction and by that we enable the patient to have convergence without active power of binocularity [40].

Similar effect has posterior fixation surgery or Faden surgery. When performing this kind of surgery, we suture the muscle to the globe at 15 mm behind the limbus and with that block the action of the muscle in the desired position [41]. Both kinds of surgeries are usually used on medial rectus muscles but can be used on other rectus muscles of the eye if we want to reduce the action of the operated muscle [42].

Nowadays we have some medications that are used for treating nystagmus (memantine, gabapentin, baclofen 4, aminopyridine, etc.), but because of a number of side effects, they are usually not used for children [43]. Some modern therapies like biofeedback (making the patients aware of the eye bobbling by sound or touch, and by that teach the patient to control nystagmus) are sometimes performed, but since there is no permanent effect, it is not widely used [44, 45].

Recently some proprioceptive nerve endings have been found at the place of the insertion of the eye muscle at the globe. Some authors advocate the idea that the cutting of the eye muscle at their insertions with reattaching or giving some medications (brinzolamide) that act on these endings can change signals and re-boost ocular motor connection and with that dampen the nystagmus [46, 47].

Conflict of interest

The authors declare no conflict of interest.

Author details

Ivana Mravicic*, Selma Lukacevic, Maja Bohac, Maja Pauk-Gulic and Vlade Glavota
Eye Clinic "Svjetlost" Medical School University of Rijeka, Zagreb, Croatia

*Address all correspondence to: ivana.mravicic@svjetlost.hr

IntechOpen

References

[1] Ehrt O. Infantile and acquired nystagmus in childhood. European Journal of Paediatric Neurology. 2012;**16**(6):567-572

[2] Abel LA. Infantile nystagmus: Current concepts in diagnosis and management. Clinical & Experimental Optometry. 2006;**89**(2):57-65

[3] CEMAS Working group. A National Eye Institute sponsored workshop and publication on the classification of the eye movement abnormalities and strabismus (CEMAS). In: The National Eye Institute Publications. Bethesda, MD: The National Eye Institutes of Health. www.nei.nih.gov.2001

[4] Nash DL, Diehl NN, Mohney BG. Incidence and Types of Pediatric Nystagmus. American Journal of Ophthalmology. 2017;**182**:31-34

[5] Sarvananthan N, Surendran M, Roberts EO, et al. The prevalence of nystagmus: The Leicestershire nystagmus survey. Investigative Ophthalmology & Visual Science. 2009; **50**:5201-5206

[6] Hertle RW, Dell'Osso LF. Clinical and ocular motor analysis of congenital nystagmus in infancy. Journal of AAPOS. 1999;**3**:70-79

[7] Kerrison JB, Koenekoop RK, Arnould VJ, Zee D, Maumenee IH. Clinical features of autosomal dominant congenital nystagmus linked to chromosome 6p12. American Journal of Ophthalmology. 1998;**125**:64-70

[8] Betts-Handerson J, Bartesaghi S, Crosier M, et al. The nystagmus-associated FRMD7 gene regulates neuronal outgrowth and development. Human Molecular Genetics. 2010;**19**: 342-351

[9] Kerrison JB, Arnould VJ, Barmada MM, et al. A gene for autosomal dominant congenital nystagmus localises to 6p12. Genomics. 1996;**33**: 523-526

[10] Ragge NK, Hartley C, Dearlove AM, et al. Familial vestibulocerebellar disorder maps to chromosome 13q31-q33: A new nystagmus locus. Journal of Medical Genetics. 2003;**40**:37-41

[11] Schlindwein P, Schreckenberger M, Dietrich M. Visual-motion suppression in congenital pendular nystagmus. Annals of the New York Academy of Sciences. 2009;**1164**:458-460. Basic and Clinical Aspects of Vertigo and Dizziness

[12] Gretsy MA, Barratt HJ, Page GR, Ell JJ. Assessment of vestibular-ocular reflexes in congenital nystagmus. American Academy of Neurology. 1985; **17**:129-136

[13] Dell's Osso LF et al. Foveation dynamics in congenital nystagmus: I. Fixation. Documenta Ophthalmologica. 1992;**79**:1-23

[14] Abadi RV, Whittle J. The nature of head postures in congenital nystagmus. Archives of Ophthalmology. 1991;**109**: 216-220

[15] Weiss AH, Biersdorf WR. Visual sensory disorders in congenital nystagmus. Ophthalmology. 1989;**96**: 517-523

[16] Pearce WG. Congenital nystagmus. Genetic and environmental causes. Canadian Journal of Ophthalmology. 1987;**13**:1-9

[17] Kanski JJ, Bowling B (2011) Congenital cataract, In: Clinical Ophthalmology: A Systematic Approach 7th ed. Elsevier Saunders, Edinburgh/

London/New York/Philadelphia/St Luis/
Toronto

[18] Hwang SS, Kim SS, Lee SJ. Clinical
features of strabismus and nystagmus in
bilateral congenital cataracts.
International Journal of Ophthalmology.
2018;**11**(5):813-817

[19] Russell HC, McDougall V, Dutton
GN. Congenital cataract. BMJ. 2011;**342**:
d3075

[20] Karim MA, Aozuki K, Fukai K, Of J,
Nagle DL, Moore KJ, et al. Apparent
genotype-phenotype correlation in
childhood, adolescent, and adult
Chediak-Higashi. American Journal of
Medical Genetics. 2002;**108**:16-22

[21] Camand O, Marchant D, Boutboul S,
Pequignot M, Odent S, Dollfus H, et al.
Mutation analysis of tyrosinase gene in
oculocutaneous albinism. Human
Mutation. 2001;**17**:352-358

[22] Levin AV, Strol EJ. Albinism for the
busy clinician. Journal of AAPOS. 2011;
15:59-66

[23] Benarroch EE. The melanopsin
system: Phototransduction, projections,
functions and clinical implications.
Neurology. 2011;**76**(16):1422-1427

[24] Hoffman MB, Lorenz B, Morland
AB, Schmidtborn LC. Misrouting of the
optic nerves in albinisms: Estimation of
the extent with visual evoked potentials.
Investigative Ophthalmology & Visual
Science. 2005;**46**(10):3892-3898

[25] Petros TJ, Rebsam A, Mason CA.
Retinal axon growth at the optic chiasm:
To cross or not to cross. Annual Review
of Neuroscience. 2008;**31**:295-315

[26] Creel D, O'Donnell FE Jr, Wukop CJ
Jr. Visual system anomalies in human
ocular albinos. Science. 1978;**201**:
931-933

[27] Preising MN, Forster H, Gonser M,
Lorenz B. Screening for TYR, OCA2,
GPR143 and MC1R in patients with
congenital nystagmus, macular
hypoplasia and fundus
hypopigmentation indicating albinism.
Molecular Vision. 2011;**17**:939-948

[28] Abadi RV, Scallan CJ. Waveform
characteristics of manifest latent
nystagmus. Investigative
Ophthalmology and Visual Science.
2000;**41**(12):3805-3817

[29] Dell'Osso LF, Schmidt D, Daroff
RB. Latent, manifest latent and
congenital nystagmus. Archives of
Ophthalmology. 1979;**97**:1877-1885

[30] Ciancia AO. Early esotropia.
International Ophthalmology Clinics.
1971;**4**:81-87

[31] Weissman BM, Dell'Osso LF, Abel
LA, Leigh RJ. Spasmus nutans. A
quantitative prospective study. Archives
of Ophthalmology. 1987;**105**(4):525-528

[32] Brodsky MC. Nystagmus in
children. In: Pediatric Neuro-
Ophthalmology. New York, NY:
Springer; 2016

[33] Anderson JR. Causes and treatment
of congenital eccentric nystagmus. The
British Journal of Ophthalmology. 1953;
37:267

[34] Kestenbaum A. Nouvelle operation
de nystagmus. Bull Soc Ophthalmol
France. 1954;**2**:1071-1078

[35] Conrad HG, De Decker W.
Torsional Kestenbaum procedure:
Evolution of a surgical concept. In:
Reinecke RD, editor. Strabismus II. New
York: Grune and Stratton; 1982. p. 301

[36] Parks MM. Congenital nystagmus
surgery. The American Orthoptic
Journal. 1973;**23**:35-39

[37] Nelson LB, Erwin-Mulley LD, Calhoun JH, Harley RD, Keisler MS. Surgical management for abnormal head position in nystagmus: The augmented modified Kestenbaum procedure. The British Journal of Ophthalmology. 1984;**68**:796-800

[38] Pratt-Johnson JA. Results of surgery to modify the null-zone position in congenital nystagmus. Canadian Journal of Ophthalmology. 1991;**26**:219-223

[39] Sedler S, Shallo-Hoffman J, Muhlendyck H. Die Artifizielle-Divergenz-Operation beim kongenitalen Nystagmus. Fortschritte der Ophthalmologie. 1990;**87**:85-89

[40] Hoeranter R, Priglinger S, Halswanter T. Reduction of ocular muscle torque by splitting of the rectus muscle II: Technique and results. The British Journal of Ophthalmology. 2004;**88**:1409-1413

[41] Leitch RJ, Burke JP, Strachan IM. Convergence excess esotropia treated surgically with fadenoperation and medial rectus recessions. The British Journal of Ophthalmology. 1990;**74**:278-279

[42] Hoerantner R, Priglinger S, Koch M, Halswanter T. A comparison of two different techniques for oculomotor torque reduction. Acta Ophthalmologica Scandinavica. 2007;**85**(7):734-738

[43] McLean R, Proudlock F, Thomas S, Degg C, Gottlob I. Congenital nystagmus:randomized, controlled, double-masked trial of memantine/gabapentin. Annals of Neurology. 2007;**61**:130-138

[44] Glasauer S, Kalla R, Buttner U, Strupp M, Brandt T. 4-aminopyridine restores visual ocular motor function in upbeat nystagmus. Journal of Neurology, Neurosurgery, and Psychiatry. 2005;**76**:451-453

[45] Sharma P et al. Reduction of congenital nystagmus amplitude with auditory biofeedback. Journal of AAPOS. 2000;**4**:287-290

[46] Hertle RW, Chan CC, Galita DA, et al. Neuroanatomy of the extraocular muscle tendon enthesis in macaque, normal human, and patients with congenital nystagmus. Journal of AAPOS. 2002;**6**(5):319-327

[47] Hertle RW, Dell'Osso LF, FitzGibbon EJ, et al. Horizontal rectus muscle tenotomy in children with infantile nystagmus syndrome: A pilot study. Journal of AAPOS. 2004;**8**(6):539-548

Chapter 5

Eye Movement Abnormalities in Neurodegenerative Diseases

Roberto Rodríguez-Labrada, Yaimeé Vázquez-Mojena and Luis Velázquez-Pérez

Abstract

Neurodegenerative disorders consist in heterogeneous group of neurological conditions characterized by a wide spectrum of clinical features resulting from a progressive involvement of distinct neuron populations. Oculomotor abnormalities take a key place in the clinical picture of these disorders because the neurodegenerative processes involve the brain circuits of eye movements. The most common abnormalities include the saccadic dysfunction, fixation instability, and abnormal smooth pursuit. The clinical assessment of oculomotor function can help to differentiate diagnosis, while electrophysiological measures provide useful biomarkers for the understanding of disease physiopathology and progression. In this chapter, we review the state of the art of the eye movement's deficits in some neurodegenerative diseases, such as Parkinson's disease, Alzheimer's disease, amyotrophic lateral sclerosis, Huntington's disease, and the hereditary ataxias.

Keywords: eye movements, oculomotor abnormalities, neurodegenerative disorders, biomarkers, Parkinson's disease, Alzheimer's disease, dementia, hereditary ataxias

1. Introduction

Neurodegenerative disorders encompass a highly heterogeneous group of complex neurological disorder characterized by progressive dysfunction and loss of neuron populations leading a wide spectrum of clinical features that cause notable motor and/or intellectual disabilities regularly incompatible with the life [1]. Consequently, some of these conditions represent important public health concern and has been identified as a research priority. Although physiopathological mechanisms generally differ among neurodegenerative diseases, a great number of them are characterized by abnormal accumulation of misfolded protein resulting in the loss of their physiological function and/or the gain of toxic functions [2, 3].

Classification of neurodegenerative disorders can be established by both the cardinal clinical features and the disease proteins (**Figure 1**). The former characterization distinguishes those conditions characterized by dementia syndromes and the movement disorders. Among dementias, the most commonly recognized disorder is the Alzheimer's disease. Other dementia syndromes include the frontotemporal dementia, the posterior cortical atrophy, the corticobasal syndrome, and others. Movement disorders comprise hypokinetic (such as Parkinson's disease) and hyperkinetic (such as Huntington's disease) conditions, as well

A

NEURODEGENERATIVE DISEASES

DEMENTIA
•*Alzheimer disease*
•*Fronto-temporal dementia*
•*Posterior cortical atrophy*
•*Corticobasal syndrome*

MOVEMENT DISORDERS

Hypokinetic movements	Hyperkinetic movements	Cerebellar Ataxias	Motoneuron diseases
•*Parkinson disease* •*Parkinsonian syndromes*	•*Huntington disease* •*Other choreas*	•*Spinocerebellar ataxias* •*Friedreich Ataxia* •*Ataxia telangiectasia*	•*Amyotrophic lateral sclerosis*

B

NEURODEGENERATIVE DISEASES

Tautopahies	a-synucleino-pathies	TDP-43 & FUS proteinopathies	Polyglutamino-pathies	Prion disease
•Alzheimer disease	•Parkinson disease •Dementia with Lewy bodies •Multisystem atrophy	•Amyotrophic lateral sclerosis •Frontotemporal lobar degeneration	•Huntington disease •Spinocerebellar ataxias 1, 2, 3, 6, 7, 17 •DRPLA •SBMA	•Creutzfeldt-Jakob disease

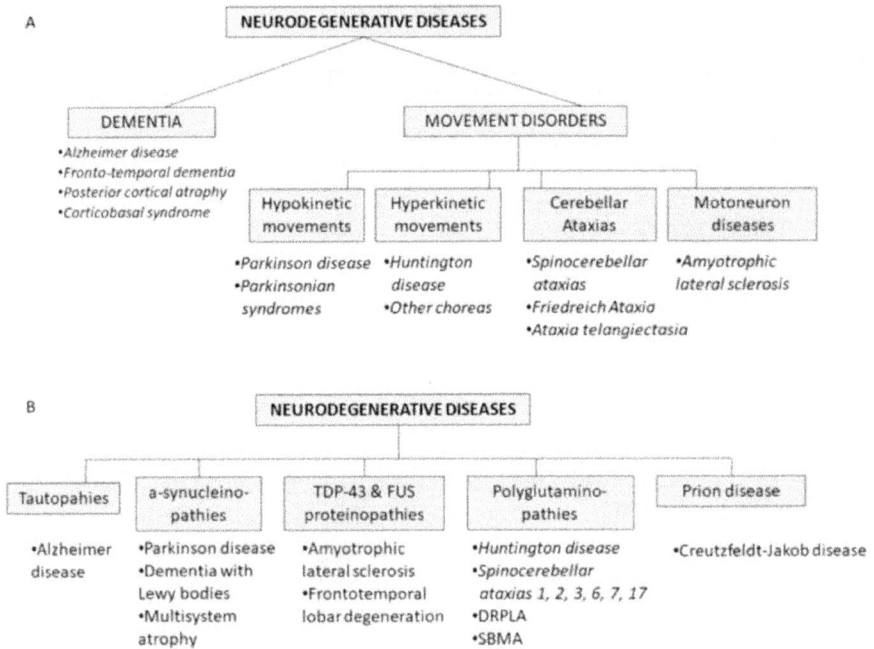

Figure 1.
Classification of neurodegenerative diseases according to cardinal syndrome (A) and disease proteins (B).

as cerebellar ataxias and motor neuron diseases (such as amyotrophic lateral sclerosis) [1, 4].

The protein-based classification includes the tauopathies, the a-synucleinopathies, the TDP-43 and FUS proteinopathies, the polyglutamine diseases, and the prion disease. Tauopathies are caused by abnormal accumulation of tau protein and B-amyloids and are represented by the Alzheimer dementia, whereas among the a-synucleinopathies are recognized as the Parkinson's disease, dementia with Lewy bodies, and multisystem atrophy. Abnormal accumulation of TDP-43 and FUS proteins defines the physiopathology of the amyotrophic lateral sclerosis and frontotemporal lobar degeneration, whereas the polyglutamine diseases result from the accumulation of proteins with abnormally expanded polyglutamine domains and include the Huntington's disease; the spinocerebellar ataxias 1, 2, 3, 6, 7, and 17; the dentatorubral-pallidoluysian atrophy; and the spinal and bulbar muscular atrophy. Finally, the Creutzfeldt-Jakob disease is classified as a prion disease [1, 4].

Although the phenotypical features of neurodegenerative disorders generally differ between distinct disorders due to the differential involvement of specific functional systems, most of these conditions are characterized by altered oculomotor function as a result of the high vulnerability of the oculomotor system to the toxic protein deposition and other physiopathological mechanisms causing neurodegenerative diseases [5, 6]. Accordingly, the assessment of oculomotor function has become a helpful approach to diagnose some of the neurodegenerative diseases. Besides, eye movements are usually used for monitoring of disease progression [6, 7].

This chapter is focused to review the state of the art of the eye movement's deficits in some neurodegenerative diseases, such as Parkinson's disease, Alzheimer's disease, amyotrophic lateral sclerosis, Huntington's disease, and the hereditary ataxias.

2. Brief overview of eye movements

Eye movements facilitate the clear vision stabilizing images on the retina, particularly against head and body movements, capturing and keeping specific stimuli on the fovea and aligning the retinal images in the two eyes to ensure the single vision and stereopsis. Ocular motility is guaranteed by five basic types of eye movements: the vestibulo-ocular reflex, the optokinetic reflex, the saccadic movements, the smooth pursuit movements, and the vergence [8].

Although they differ in various aspects, such as their velocity, reaction time, reflexivity/volitional degree, and their neurobiological substrates [9], all have generic kinematic properties and share a common final path represented by three cranial nerve nuclei and the three pairs of eye muscles that they control [8, 10]. Cranial nerve III (oculomotor) innervates the superior, inferior, and medial rectus muscles as well as the inferior oblique muscle, whereas trochlear (IV) and abducens (VI) nerves innervate the superior oblique and lateral rectus, respectively [10].

The vestibulo-ocular reflex (VOR) is elicited by the vestibular system in response to body/head rotations and consists on compensatory eye movements in opposite direction to body/head movements to guarantee the image stabilization on the retina [11]. When head/body rotations are very large and continued, the VOR is depressed, and thus, it is complemented by the optokinetic reflex (OKR), in which the speed and direction of a full-field image motion are computed to develop eye movements with two phases: a slow phase that alternates with resetting a quick phase [12].

Saccades are ballistic and conjugate eye movements that redirect the fovea from one object of interest to another, allowing to explore accurately the visual scenes. For that, saccadic system processes information about the distance and direction of a target image from the current position of gaze. Saccades are the fastest eye movements, reaching up to 800/s. Behaviorally, saccades may be classified as reflex-guided saccades and intentional or volitional saccades. The first ones are evoked by suddenly appearing targets, whereas the second ones, called also as higher-order saccades, are made purposefully. Therefore, intentional saccades involve high-cognitive processing and include voluntary, memory-guided and delayed saccades, as well as antisaccades [13, 14].

Smooth pursuit eye movements enable us to maintain the image of a moving object relatively stable on or near the fovea by matching eye velocity to target velocity [10]. Smooth pursuit performance is optimal for target speeds ranging between 150/s and 300/s, but pursuit velocity can reach up to 100/s [8, 15].

Vergence eye movements are disjunctive movements that provide the binocular alignment in response to changing fixation of target distances, requiring that both eyes point in contrary directions. These movements are elicited by retinal disparity (when a fixation target is not on both foveae) and retinal blur (when a target is not in focus). Therefore, these movements are closely related to the lens accommodation and pupillary reflexes [16].

3. Oculomotor disturbances in neurodegenerative diseases

3.1 Parkinson's disease and other parkinsonian disorders

3.1.1 Parkinson's disease

Parkinson's disease is a progressive disorder pathologically defined by the degeneration of the dopaminergic neurons in the *substantia nigra* and formation of α-synuclein-containing Lewy bodies in the residual dopaminergic neurons. Consequently, the clinical picture is characterized by progressive motor symptoms that include bradykinesia, muscular rigidity, rest tremor, as well as postural and gait impairment. The disease is also associated with many non-motor symptoms, some of which precede the motor dysfunction by more than a decade [17]. Global prevalence of PD ranges between 100 and 200 cases per 100,000 inhabitants, with an annual incidence around 15 cases per 100,000 [18]. Although the etiology of PD is commonly unknown, monogenic causes can be considered in 5–10% of the cases [19].

Findings about oculomotor function in PD are certainly inconsistent due to the reduced number of patients included in the majority of the studies and the heterogeneity of the disease phenotype [7]. Nevertheless, saccadic hypometria is recognized as the most striking oculomotor feature in PD patients, which can be documented both at bedside and by electrophysiological approaches even early in the disease course. As a result of the saccade hypometria, PD patients frequently require multistep sequences to reach the target [20]. This behavior is more pronounced during memory-guided saccades, and it is considered as a disease biomarker [21, 22]. The marked saccade hypometria in PD can be explained by the neurodegenerative changes in the basal ganglia causing the decrease of pre-oculomotor drive through the substantia nigra to the superior colliculus [21]. Alongside the saccade hypometria, PD patients also show abnormally prolonged latency of voluntary saccades such as the memory-guided saccades and the antisaccades; nevertheless, the latency of externally triggered saccades to visual targets is normal [23]. Distinct to the saccade hypometria, the deficits in the saccade initiation are detectable later in the disease course and are closely related with the cognitive impairments and the involvement of non-dopaminergic pathways such as the frontal and parietal eye fields, the premotor cortex, and the lateral prefrontal cortex [24].

The delayed prosaccade and the antisaccade tasks reveal an impaired inhibition of saccades as evidence of deficit of automatic response inhibition. PD patients show increased timing error rates in the delayed prosaccade paradigm, which are closely associated with abnormal neuropsychological performance, whereas antisaccade paradigm reveals higher directional error rates [25]. Antisaccade errors can be detected early in the disease course [26]. Beyond saccadic impairments, PD patients show slight alterations in other eye movements, such as reduced gain of the smooth pursuit movements [27] and slow and hypometric divergence movements, but normal convergence movements [28].

3.1.2 Other parkinsonian disorders

Oculomotor findings of patients suffering from other parkinsonian disorders are varied and usually distinctive to the PD. In cases with multisystem atrophy with predominant Parkinsonism (MSA-P), the clinical assessments of oculomotor function usually reveal increased square wave jerks, saccade hypometria, as well as abnormal smooth pursuit and vestibulo-ocular reflex [29, 30]. Less common oculomotor features in MSA-P include downbeat nystagmus, head-shaking nystagmus, and mild vertical supranuclear gaze palsy [29, 31].

In the progressive supranuclear palsy with Parkinsonism (PSP-P), the most important oculomotor feature is the slowing of vertical saccades, which progresses to supranuclear gaze palsy in the 70% of the cases but appear lately in the disease course than in the classic PSP [32]. In addition, these patients show reduced gains of the smooth pursuit movements and saccadic eye movements at similar extent that in classic PSP [27].

3.2 Alzheimer's disease and other dementias

3.2.1 Alzheimer's disease

Alzheimer's disease (AD) is the most common neurodegenerative disorder worldwide with a global prevalence above 20 million of affected people, which is estimated to grow notably in the next decades. The histopathological hallmark of the disease is the deposition of insoluble protein aggregates such as amyloid-β (Aβ) plaques and neurofibrillary tangles of tau in the brain, causing a significant brain atrophy and subsequent cognitive features such as memory disturbances, executive dysfunction, difficulties with language, and other cognitive skills that affect a person's ability to perform every day [33]. Similar to PD, the etiology of Alzheimer's disease (AD) is not fully understood, but several environmental and genetic factors are assumed to contribute to the disease etiopathogenesis [34].

Oculomotor testing in Alzheimer's disease reveals a varied group of eye movement abnormalities, but no specific oculomotor feature is distinguished. Among oculomotor features of AD patients, the saccadic intrusions are one of the most common [35, 36]. These unwanted microsaccades are mainly oblique and can be detected even in subjects with mild cognitive impairment which identify this oculomotor feature as a potential biomarker of Alzheimer's disease at early stages [37]. These microsaccades are more frequent in those patients with higher dementia scores [38], which support the notion that gaze-fixation instability in AD results from the involvement of cognitive processes such as the attention and working memory. Nevertheless, the impairment of the saccade pathways could also explain the high occurrence of saccadic intrusions, mainly at later disease stages [39].

Reflexive and voluntary saccades of AD patients are usually characterized by prolonged latencies, reduced velocity, and hypometria. Antisaccadic paradigm reveals increased directional error rate alongside with the reduction of the error correction, which are closely associated with the severity of dementia [40]. Both prosaccadic and antisaccadic alterations in AD are proposed to result from impaired inhibitory control and attentional failures, as well as from the later involvement of saccadic circuitry at brainstem [39]. In addition, AD patients show increased latency to initiate smooth pursuit movements, with decreased gain velocity and increased catch-up (compensatory) saccades. Similar to the saccadic intrusions and antisaccadic deficits, the rate of compensatory saccades during the smooth pursuit is narrowly related with the dementia severity [40–42].

3.2.2 Other dementias

In the posterior cortical atrophy (PCA), an atypical variant of AD, the most frequent oculomotor abnormalities include increased saccade latency and decreased saccade amplitude, but the saccade velocity is normal. Also, the PCA patients show increased time to saccadic target fixation, even higher than subjects with typical AD. Moreover, these patients show large saccadic intrusions whose frequency is correlated with generalized reductions in cortical thickness. Smooth pursuit gain is slightly reduced in these patients [43, 44]. Moreover, individuals with frontotemporal dementia (FTD) show increased reflexive saccade latency and higher rates of antisaccadic errors, but the error correction abilities are preserved. In addition, the smooth pursuit movements are characterized by the reduction of gains and accelerations [40, 45, 46].

3.3 Huntington's disease

Huntington's disease is a neurodegenerative disorder caused by the abnormal expansion of cytosine-adenine-guanine (CAG) trinucleotide repeats in the huntingtin gene on chromosome 4, encoding the huntingtin protein. The mutation results in an excessively long polyglutamine stretch near the N-terminus of this protein, which identify this disorder as a polyglutamine disease. Mutant HTT affects some cellular processes, including protein-protein interaction, protein clearance, mitochondrial function, axonal trafficking, gene transcription, posttranslational modification, and others that ultimately cause the loss of striatal neurons [47].

Clinically, the disease is characterized by a progressive motor, cognitive, and psychiatric disturbance. The motor phenotype includes chorea as cardinal feature, as well as dystonia and Parkinsonism, whereas the cognitive dysfunction comprises dysexecutive signs, as well as memory and attentional dysfunction. Psychiatric features are usually depression, anxiety, apathy, obsessive-compulsive behaviors, and others. Similar to other polyglutamine disorders, the age at onset of HD is highly influenced by the CAG repeat length, but other genetic and environmental modifying factors are proposed to also control the age at onset variability [47, 48].

Oculomotor abnormalities of patients with HD include saccade slowing and deficits in the initiation and suppression of these movements. The reduction of saccade velocity appears in around 60% of patients and is commonly observed in the vertical plane, but in those cases in advanced disease stages, the saccade slowing reaches also the horizontal movements [49, 50]. Saccade latencies are significantly prolonged and show a marked variability, which is more pronounced in patients showing higher disease severity. Studies using the antisaccadic paradigm have revealed and increased rate of directional errors, which are also closely correlated with the severity of the disease. Moreover, increases of latency variability and timing errors are observed in the memory-guided saccade task. The deficits of the suppression and initiation of the saccades can be explained by the neurodegenerative changes in the frontal cortex and in the basal ganglia [51, 52]. So, a recent imaging research revealed a close association between the voluntary saccade inhibition deficits and the white-matter corticobasal atrophy in patients [53].

Several authors have evaluated saccadic eye movements in asymptomatic carriers of the HD mutation. These studies have found a significant delay in the initiation of voluntary eye movements, increase in the variability of saccadic latency, and increase in the rate of antisaccadic errors [54–56]. A longitudinal follow-up of these alterations demonstrated their usefulness as preclinical markers due to the high replicability and consistency of these measures [22]. Imaging studies in asymptomatic carriers of HD have shown a significant correspondence between alterations in saccadic latency and the decrease in the number of fronto-striatal fibers that project into the caudate nucleus and the atrophy of gray matter in cortical structures, which deepens in the pathophysiology of saccadic alterations in this disease [57, 58]. A recent paper demonstrated that the horizontal ocular pursuit item of the Unified Huntington's Disease Rating Scale is useful for detecting differences between premanifest individuals and controls [59].

3.4 Amyotrophic lateral sclerosis

Amyotrophic lateral sclerosis (ALS) is the most common and devastating age-related motor neuron disease, characterized by a progressive loss of upper and lower motoneurons, causing paralysis and death in approximately 3 years. The pathological hallmark of ALS is the presence of abundant cytoplasmic inclusions containing ubiquitin and TDP-43, a RNA-binding protein. The clinical picture comprises progressive muscle weakness alongside hyperreflexia and spasticity associated with fibrillations and fasciculations [60]. The disease has a global prevalence around five cases per 100,000 inhabitants. Most of ALS cases are sporadic, and only the 5% of patients are familial, with at least 12 genes implicated, such as the superoxide dismutase 1(SOD1), trans-activate response DNA-binding protein (TARDBP), C9ORF72, FUS, and the ataxin-2 genes [61, 62].

Some evidences have demonstrated the involvement of the oculomotor system in ALS, leading a broad range of eye movement deficits affecting the saccades and the smooth pursuit movements [63–66]. The most prominent and early oculomotor alterations of ALS patients are related with abnormal executive oculomotor control as evidence of frontal lobe involvement. They primarily includes the increase of error rates in anti-saccades and delayed saccade paradigms as well as reduced voluntary gaze shift and increased number of saccadic intrusions. In general, these oculomotor alterations are correlated with the severity of the disease and the neurocognitive measures. In a following stage of oculomotor abnormalities, some ALS cases can show slow saccades, saccade hypometria, and interrupted smooth pursuit, as evidences of the involvement of the brainstem and pre-cerebellar/pontine circuits [67].

3.5 Hereditary ataxias

Hereditary ataxias consist in a heterogeneous group of genetic disorders phenotypically characterized by gait ataxia, limb incoordination, dysmetria, dysarthria, oculomotor disturbances, and other motor and non-motor features. These disorders are associated with atrophy of the cerebellum, which can be accompanied with the degeneration of other regions in the central and peripheral nervous system in various genetic subtypes [68].

Hereditary ataxias are classified into four main groups regarding their inheritance patterns: autosomal dominant (also referred as spinocerebellar ataxias), autosomal recessive, X-linked, and mitochondrial ataxias [68, 69]. Till now, 46 subtypes of spinocerebellar ataxias have been identified, which imply at least 37 distinct genes [70]. The most common subtypes are caused by polyglutamine (polyQ)-coding CAG repeat expansions (SCA1,2,3,6,7,17, DRPLA) [71]. Regarding the recessive ataxias, nearly 100 genes have been identified, with the highest prevalence for the Friedreich's ataxia (FRDA), caused by GAA repeat expansions or point mutations in the frataxin (FXN) [68, 72]. Global prevalence of hereditary ataxias is estimated around three cases per 100,000 inhabitants, but there are large regional variations of prevalence due to founder effects of some genes [73].

Oculomotor disturbances of SCA patients are varied and result from the cerebellar and/or brainstem involvement. The former abnormalities are the most common and include the presence of pathological nystagmus, abnormal smooth pursuit, and saccadic dysmetria, whereas the impaired VOR, saccadic slowing, and ophthalmoplegia are related with pontine degeneration. Nevertheless, the notable overlapping of oculomotor features between SCA subtypes implies the requirement of other clinical criteria or the genetic testing for sensitively discriminating among these diseases [74–78] (**Figure 2**).

In the case of SCA2, an early and severe saccadic slowing is observed even more than a decade before the ataxia onset [79], which identifies it as important preclinical biomarker of the disease. Interestingly, the SCA2 saccade slowing is tightly influenced by the expanded CAG repeats in the ATXN2 gene [80] and shows a significant familiar aggregation which leads to the suitability of this disease feature as endophenotype marker [81], with potential usefulness for the search of modifier genes and neurobiological underpinnings of the disease and as outcome measure

Oculomotor
cerebellar signs

Oculomotor
brainstem signs

SCA5
SCA8
SCA11

SCA1

SCA12
SCA23
SCA25
SCA28
SCA30

SCA6

SCA2

SCA13
SCA14
SCA15/16

SCA22
SCA26
SCA36

SCA17

SCA7

SCA3

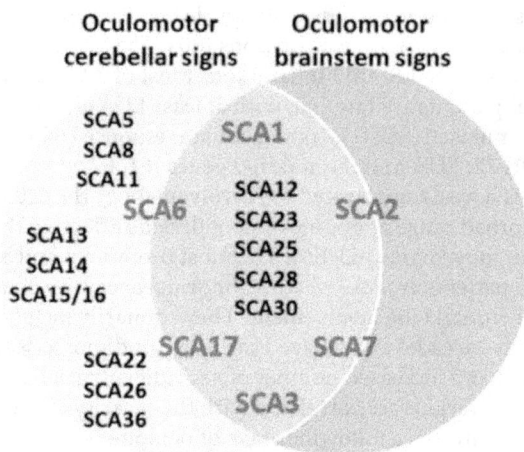

Figure 2.
Cerebellar and/or brainstem origin of oculomotor features in SCAs.

in future neuroprotective clinical trials. Moreover, the saccade slowing in SCA2 progresses significantly along time providing novel insight into the cumulative polyglutamine neurotoxicity and supporting the usefulness of saccade peak velocity as a sensitive biomarker during the natural history of the disease [82]. Saccade pathology in SCA2 is also characterized by abnormal prolongation of reflexive and voluntary latencies and increases of the antisaccade error rate. The later feature is also detected in prodromal stage and is significantly correlated with the mutation size [83–85].

The main eye movement abnormalities of SCA1 patients include saccadic dysmetria, gaze-evoked nystagmus, and depressed smooth pursuit [86]. Saccadic hypermetria is observed in majority of cases, appears at an early stage of the disease, and progresses quickly [75, 76, 87]. SCA3 is characterized by a higher frequency of gaze-evoked and rebound nystagmus [88], in addition to decreased smooth pursuit gain and saccadic dysmetria. These patients also show decreased VOR gain, which correlated with the CAG repeats, suggesting the pathologic involvement of the vestibular nuclei in the lateral brainstem [74–76]. Divergence insufficiency and strabismus are also common oculomotor features of these patients [89, 90].

In SCA6, a higher frequency of spontaneous downbeat nystagmus and square wave jerks is detected [76, 91, 92]. The square wave jerks together with subtle abnormalities of saccades and smooth pursuit movements can be detected even before the disease onset [93]. The major saccadic alteration in SCA7 is the slowing of saccades, together with saccadic dysmetria [94, 95]. These alterations may precede cerebellar and retinal manifestations by some years [96]. Patients with SCA17 show hypometric saccades which are increased with disease duration but neither with ataxia score nor CAG repeats number [97].

Eye movement disturbances are frequent in FRDA. The most prominent abnormalities consist in fixation instability such as multiple square wave jerks and ocular flutter, which are also complemented by abnormal smooth pursuit, saccadic dysmetria, prolongation of saccade latency, gaze-evoked nystagmus, and impaired VOR. Interestingly, the prolongation of saccade latency and the square wave jerks are significantly correlated with the disease severity and age at disease onset, respectively [98, 99]. Moreover, antisaccades and memory-guided saccades are also abnormal in these patients as evidence of the disruption of the higher-order processes controlling the saccade movements [100].

4. Concluding remarks

Eye movement abnormalities are among the most common phenotypic manifestations of patients with neurodegenerative diseases. The prominent features include the saccadic abnormalities, fixation instability, and abnormal smooth pursuit. Thus, the examination of eye movements is a very useful, but not determinant, approach for the differential diagnosis of these disorders. For example, the increased square wave jerks and the slowing of vertical saccades may be useful features for the clinicians in order to distinguish between the MSA-P and the PSP-P from the idiopathic Parkinson's disease, respectively. In addition, the early and severe saccadic slowing with rare pathological nystagmus distinguishes SCA2 from other autosomal dominant ataxias, whereas the marked abnormalities of smooth pursuit, VOR and OKR, in association with pathological nystagmus and rare saccadic slowing may help to define a SCA6 phenotype. Nonetheless, the notable overlapping of oculomotor features between neurodegenerative disorders suggests the necessity of other diagnostic criteria for sensitively discriminating among diseases with similar symptomatology.

Besides, the assessment of oculomotor function in neurodegenerative disorders leads to the identification of disease biomarkers, which acquire key values in the clinical and research practice of neurodegenerations. Many eye movement markers of neurodegenerative disorders allow to assess the disease stage and disease progression, because their changes over time are significantly linked with clinical outcome of syndrome severity, and interestingly some oculomotor disturbances precede the clinical diagnosis of the disease, which identify them as useful preclinical markers to detect the early stages of the neurodegenerative process, to evaluate the genetic susceptibility of the asymptomatic relatives, and to identify individuals for enrolment in early intervention trials.

Moreover, the study of eye movements in neurodegenerative diseases offers valuable advantages to assess the cognitive functioning in these conditions, mainly those measures that reflect the high-order processes underlying the oculomotor functions such as the antisaccade and memory-guided saccade task outcomes, the saccade latency, and others.

In conclusion, although by decades the oculomotor system has been widely studied in neurodegenerative diseases, further efforts are warranted to study their involvement in other—less common—disorders, to understand the physiopathological mechanisms underlying oculomotor disturbances and to certify the role of oculomotor features as sensitive outcome measures in further neuroprotective trials.

Acknowledgements

We are very indebted to Cuban Ministry of Public Health for their collaboration.

Conflict of interest

Authors declared no conflict of interest.

Appendices and nomenclature

AD	Alzheimer's disease
ALS	amyotrophic lateral sclerosis

CAG	cytosine-adenine-guanine trinucleotide
DRPLA	dentatorubral-pallidoluysian atrophy
FRDA	Friedreich's ataxia
FTD	frontotemporal dementia
FXN	frataxin
HD	Huntington's disease
MSA-P	multisystem atrophy with predominant Parkinsonism
OKR	optokinetic reflex
PCA	posterior cortical atrophy
PD	Parkinson's disease
PSP-P	progressive supranuclear palsy with Parkinsonism
SCA	spinocerebellar ataxia
VOR	vestibulo-ocular reflex

Author details

Roberto Rodríguez-Labrada[1*], Yaimeé Vázquez-Mojena[1] and Luis Velázquez-Pérez[1,2]

1 Centre for the Research and Rehabilitation of Hereditary Ataxias, Holguin, Cuba

2 Cuban Academy of Sciences, Havana, Cuba

*Address all correspondence to: robertrl1981@gmail.com

IntechOpen

References

[1] Kovacs GG. Concepts and classification of neurodegenerative diseases. Handbook of Clinical Neurology. 2017;**145**:302-307

[2] Carrell RW, Lomas DA. Conformational disease. Lancet. 1997;**350**:134-138

[3] Csizmok V, Tompa P. Structural disorder and its connection with misfolding diseases. In: Ovadi J, Orosz F, editors. Protein Folding and Misfolding: Neurodegenerative Diseases, Focus on Structural Biology. Vol. 7. Dordrecht: Springer; 2009. pp. 1-20. ISBN: 978-1-4020-9433-0

[4] Kovacs GG. Classification of neurodegenerative diseases. In: Kovacs GG, editor. Neuropathology of Neurodegenerative Diseases: A Practical Guide. Cambridge: Cambridge University Press; 2016. pp. 1-7. ISBN: 978-1-107-44242-9

[5] MacAskill MR, Anderson TJ. Eye movements in neurodegenerative diseases. Current Opinion in Neurology. 2016;**29**:61-68

[6] Gorges M, Pinkhardt EH, Kassubek J. Alterations of eye movement control in neurodegenerative movement disorders. Journal of Ophthalmology. 2014;**2014**:658243

[7] Anderson TJ, MacAskill MR. Eye movements in patients with neurodegenerative disorders. Nature Reviews Neurology. 2013;**9**:74-85

[8] Bruce CH, Friedman HR. Eye movements. Encyclopedia of the Human Brain. 2002;**2**:269-297

[9] Sparks DL. The brainstem control of saccadic eye movements. Nature Reviews Neuroscience. 2002;**3**:952-964

[10] Leigh RJ, Zee DS. The Neurology of Eye Movements. 4th ed. New York, USA: Oxford University Press; 2006

[11] Aw ST, Haslwanter T, Halmagyi GM, Curthoys IS, Yavor RA, Todd MJ. Three-dimensional vector analysis of the human vestibuloocular reflex in response to high-acceleration head rotations. I. Responses in normal subjects. Journal of Neurophysiology. 1996;**76**:4009-4020

[12] Tusa R, Zee D. Cerebral control of smooth pursuit and optokinetic nystagmus. Current Opinion in Ophthalmology. 1989;**2**:115-146

[13] Müri RM, Nyffeler T. Neurophysiology and neuroanatomy of reflexive and volitional saccades as revealed by lesion studies with neurological patients and transcranial magnetic stimulation (TMS). Brain and Cognition. 2008;**68**:284-292

[14] Leigh RJ, Kennard C. Using saccades as a research tool in the clinical neurosciences. Brain. 2004;**127**:460-477. ISSN 1460-2156

[15] Lencer R, Trillenberg P. Neurophysiology and neuroanatomy of smooth pursuit in humans. Brain and Cognition. 2008;**68**:219-228

[16] Zee DS, Levi L. Neurological aspects of vergence eye movements. Revista de Neurologia. 1989;**145**:613-620

[17] Kalia LV, Lang AE. Parkinson's disease. Lancet. 2015;**386**:896-912

[18] Tysnes OB, Storstein A. Epidemiology of Parkinson's disease. Journal of Neural Transmission (Vienna). 2017;**124**(8):901-905

[19] Singleton AB, Farrer MJ, Bonifati V. The genetics of Parkinson's disease: Progress and therapeutic implications. Movement Disorders. 2013;**28**:14-23

[20] DeJong JD, Jones GM. Akinesia, hypokinesia, and bradykinesia in the oculomotor system of patients with Parkinson's disease. Experimental Neurology. 1971;**32**:58-68

[21] Kimmig H, Haussmann K, Mergner T, Lucking CH. What is pathological with gaze shift fragmentation in Parkinson's disease? Journal of Neurology. 2002;**249**: 683-692

[22] Blekher T, Weaver M, Rupp J, Nichols WC, Hui SL, Gray J, et al. Multiple step pattern as a biomarker in Parkinson disease. Parkinsonism & Related Disorders. 2009;**15**:506-510

[23] Terao Y, Fukuda H, Ugawa Y, Hikosaka O. New perspectives on the pathophysiology of Parkinson's disease as assessed by saccade performance: A clinical review. Clinical Neurophysiology. 2013;**124**(8):1491-1506

[24] Perneczky R, Ghosh BC, Hughes L, Carpenter RH, Barker RA, Rowe JB. Saccadic latency in Parkinson's disease correlates with executive function and brain atrophy, but not motor severity. Neurobiology of Disease. 2011;**43**:79-85

[25] van Stockum S, MacAskill MR, Anderson TJ, Dalrymple-Alford JC. Don't look now or look away: Two sources of saccadic disinhibition in Parkinson's disease? Neuropsychologia. 2008;**46**:3108-3115

[26] Antoniades CA, Demeyere N, Kennard C, et al. Antisaccades and executive dysfunction in early drug-naive Parkinson's disease: The discovery study. Movement Disorders. 2015;**30**:843-847

[27] Pinkhardt EH, Jürgens R, Lulé D, Heimrath J, Ludolph AC, Becker W, et al. Eye movement impairments in Parkinson's disease: Possible role of extradopaminergic mechanisms. BMC Neurology. 2012;**12**:2-8

[28] Hanuska J, Bonnet C, Rusz J, et al. Fast vergence eye movements are disrupted in Parkinson's disease: A video-oculography study. Parkinsonism & Related Disorders. 2015;**21**:797-799

[29] Anderson T, Luxon L, Quinn N, Daniel S, David Marsden C, Bronstein A. Oculomotor function in multiple system atrophy: Clinical and laboratory features in 30 patients. Movement Disorders. 2008;**23**:977-984

[30] Linder J, Wenngren BI, Stenlund H, Forsgren L. Impaired oculomotor function in a community-based patient population with newly diagnosed idiopathic parkinsonism. Journal of Neurology. 2012;**259**:1206-1214

[31] Lee JY, Lee WW, Kim JS, Kim HJ, Kim JK, Jeon BS. Perverted head-shaking and positional downbeat nystagmus in patients with multiple system atrophy. Movement Disorders. 2009;**24**:1290-1295

[32] Williams DR et al. Characteristics of two distinct clinical phenotypes in pathologically proven progressive supranuclear palsy: Richardson's syndrome and PSP-parkinsonism. Brain. 2005;**128**:1247-1258

[33] Ballard C, Gauthier S, Brayne C, Aarsland D, Jones E. Alzheimer's disease. Lancet. 2011;**377**:1019-1031

[34] Jiang T, Yu JT, Tian Y, Tan L. Epidemiology and etiology of Alzheimer's disease: From genetic to non-genetic factors. Current Alzheimer Research. 2013;**10**:852-867

[35] Jones A, Friedland RP, Koss B, Stark L, Thompkins-Ober BA. Saccadic intrusions in Alzheimer-type dementia. Journal of Neurology. 1983;**229**: 189-194

[36] Fletcher WA, Sharpe JA. Saccadic eye movement dysfunction in Alzheimer's disease. Annals of Neurology. 1986;**20**:464-471

[37] Kapoula Z, Yang Q, Otero-Millan J, et al. Distinctive features of microsaccades in Alzheimer's disease and in mild cognitive impairment. Age. 2014;**36**:535-543

[38] Bylsma FW, Rasmusson DX, Rebok GW, Keyl PM, Tune L, Brandt J. Changes in visual fixation and saccadic eye movements in Alzheimer's disease. International Journal of Psychophysiology. 1995;**19**:33-40

[39] Parvizi J, Van Hoesen GW, Damasio A. The selective vulnerability of brainstem nuclei to Alzheimer's disease. Annals of Neurology. 2001;**49**:53-66

[40] Garbutt S, Matlin A, Hellmuth J, Schenk AK, Johnson JK, Rosen H, et al. Oculomotor function in frontotemporal lobar degeneration, related disorders and Alzheimer's disease. Brain. 2008;**131**:1268-1281

[41] Shafiq-Antonacci R, Maruff P, Masters C, Currie J. Spectrum of saccade system function in Alzheimer disease. Archives of Neurology. 2003;**60**:1272-1278

[42] Yang Q, Wang T, Su N, Liu Y, Xiao S, Kapoula Z. Long latency and high variability in accuracy-speed of prosaccades in Alzheimer's disease at mild to moderate stage. Dementia and Geriatric Cognitive Disorders Extra. 2011;**1**:318-329

[43] Shakespeare TJ, Kaski D, Yong KX, Paterson RW, Slattery CF, Ryan NS, et al. Brain. Abnormalities of fixation, saccade and pursuit in posterior cortical atrophy. 2015;**138**(Pt 7):1976-1991

[44] Suarez Gonzalez A, Henley SM, Walton J, Crutch SJ. Posterior cortical atrophy: An atypical variant of Alzheimer disease. The Psychiatric Clinics of North America. 2015;**38**:211-220

[45] Meyniel C, Rivaud-Pechoux S, Damier P, Gaymard B. Saccade impairments in patients with fronto-temporal dementia. Journal of Neurology, Neurosurgery, and Psychiatry. 2005;**76**:1581-1584

[46] Boxer AL, Garbutt S, Seeley WW, Jafari A, Heuer HW, Mirsky J, et al. Saccade abnormalities in autopsy-confirmed frontotemporal lobar degeneration and Alzheimer's disease. Archives of Neurology. 2012;**69**:509-517

[47] Bates GP, Dorsey R, Gusella JF, Hayden MR, Kay C, Leavitt BR, et al. Huntington disease. Nature Reviews. Disease Primers. 2015;**1**:15005. DOI: 10.1038/nrdp.2015.5

[48] Kim SD, Fung VS. An update on Huntington's disease: From the gene to the clinic. Current Opinion in Neurology. 2014;**27**:477-483. DOI: 10.1097/WCO.0000000000000116

[49] Leigh RJ, Newman SA, Folstein SE, Lasker AG, Jensen BA. Abnormal ocular motor control in Huntington's disease. Neurology. 1983;**33**:1268-1275

[50] Lasker AG, Zee DS, Hain TC, Folstein SE, Singer HS. Saccades in Huntington's disease. Slowing and dysmetria. Neurology. 1998;**38**:427-431

[51] Peltsch A, Hoffman A, Armstrong I, Pari G, Munoz DP. Saccadic impairments in Huntington's disease. Experimental Brain Research. 2008;**186**:457-469

[52] Patel SS, Jankovic J, Hood AJ, Jeter CB, Sereno AB. Reflexive and volitional saccades: Biomarkers of Huntington disease severity and progression. Journal of the Neurological Sciences. 2012;**203**:35-41

[53] Vaca-Palomares I, Coea BC, Brien DC, Munoz DP, Fernandez-Ruiz J. Voluntary saccade inhibition deficits correlate with extended white-matter cortico-basal atrophy in Huntington's disease. NeuroImage: Clinical. 2017;**15**:502-512

[54] Blekher T, Johnson SA, Marshall J, White K, Hui S, Weaver M, et al. Saccades in presymptomatic and early stages of Huntington disease. Neurology. 2006;**67**:394-399

[55] Golding CV, Danchaivijitr C, Hodgson TL, Tabrizi SJ, Kennard C. Identification of an oculomotor biomarker of preclinical Huntington disease. Neurology. 2006;**67**:485-487

[56] Antoniades CA, Altham PM, Mason SL, Barker RA, Carpenter R. Saccadometry: A new tool for evaluating presymptomatic Huntington patients. Neuroreport. 2007;**18**:1133-1136

[57] Kloppel S, Draganski B, Golding CV, Chu C, Nagy Z, Cook PA, et al. White matter connections reflect changes in voluntary-guided saccades in pre-symptomatic Huntington's disease. Brain. 2008;**131**(Pt 1):196-204

[58] Rupp J, Dzemidzic M, Blekher T, West J, Hui S, Wojcieszek J, et al. Comparison of vertical and horizontal saccade measures and their relation to gray matter changes in premanifest and manifest Huntington disease. Journal of Neurology. 2012;**259**:267-276

[59] Winder JY, Roos RA. Premanifest Huntington's disease: Examination of oculomotor abnormalities in clinical practice. PLoS One. 2018;**13**:e0193866

[60] Wijesekera LC, Leigh PN. Amyotrophic lateral sclerosis. Orphanet Journal of Rare Diseases. 2009;**4**:3

[61] Byrne S, Walsh C, Lynch C, et al. Rate of familial amyotrophic lateral sclerosis: A systematic review and meta-analysis. Journal of Neurology, Neurosurgery, and Psychiatry. 2011;**82**:623-627

[62] Andersen PM, Al-Chalabi A. Clinical genetics of amyotrophic lateral sclerosis: What do we really know? Nature Reviews. Neurology. 2011;**7**:603-615

[63] Jacobs L, Bozian D, Heffner RR Jr, Barron SA. An eye movement disorder in amyotrophic lateral sclerosis. Neurology. 1981;**31**:1282-1287

[64] Averbuch-Heller L, Helmchen C, Horn AK, Leigh RJ, Buttner-Ennerver JA. Slow vertical saccades in motor neuron disease: Correlation of structure and function. Annals of Neurology. 1998;**44**:641-648

[65] Donaghy C, Pinnock R, Abrahams S, et al. Slow saccades in bulbar-onset motor neurone disease. Journal of Neurology. 2010;**257**:1134-1140

[66] Sharma R, Hicks S, Berna CM, Kennard C, Talbot K, Turner MR. Oculomotor dysfunction in amyotrophic lateral sclerosis. A comprehensive review. Archives of Neurology. 2011;**68**:857-861

[67] Gorges M, Müller HP, Lulé D, Del Tredici K, Pfandl K, Ludolph AC, et al. Eye movement deficits are consistent with a staging model of pTDP-43 pathology in amyotrophic lateral sclerosis. PLoS One. 2012;**10**:e0142546

[68] Hersheson J, Haworth A, Houlden H. The inherited ataxias: Genetic heterogeneity, mutation databases, and future directions in research and clinical diagnostics. Human Mutation. 2012;**33**(9):1324-1332

[69] Mancuso M, Orsucci D, Bonuccell U. The genetics of ataxia: Through the labyrinth of the minotaur, looking for Ariadne's thread. Journal of Neurology. 2014;**261**(Suppl 2):S528-S541

[70] Ashizawa T, Öz G, Paulson HL. Spinocerebellar ataxias: Prospects and challenges for therapy development. Nature Reviews Neurology. 2018;**14**(10):590-605. DOI: 10.1038/s41582-018-0051-6

[71] Paulson HL, Shakkottai VG, Clark B, Orr HT. Polyglutamine spinocerebellar ataxias—From genes to potential treatments. Nature Reviews. Neuroscience. 2017;**18**(10):613-626

[72] Anheim M, Tranchant C, Koenig M. The autosomal recessive cerebellar ataxias. New England Journal of Medicine. 2012;**366**:636-646

[73] Ruano L, Melo C, Silva MC, Coutinho P. The global epidemiology of hereditary ataxia and spastic paraplegia: A systematic review of prevalence studies. Neuroepidemiology. 2014;**42**:174-183. DOI: 10.1159/000358801

[74] Burk K, Fetter M, Abele M, Laccone F, Brice A, Dichgans J, et al. Autosomal dominant cerebellar ataxia type I: Oculomotor abnormalities in families with SCA1, SCA2, and SCA3. Journal of Neurology. 1999;**246**:789-797. ISSN 0340-5354

[75] Rivaud-Pechoux S, Durr A, Gaymard B, Cancel G, Ploner CJ, Agid Y, et al. Eye movement abnormalities correlate with genotype in autosomal dominant cerebellar ataxia type I. Annals of Neurology. 1998;**43**:297-302. ISSN 1531-8249

[76] Buttner JA, Geschwind D, Jen JC, Perlman S, Pulst SM, Baloh RW. Oculomotor phenotypes in autosomal dominant ataxias. Archives of Neurology. 1998;**55**:1353-1357. ISSN 1538-3687

[77] Rodríguez-Labrada R, Velazquez-Perez L. Eye movement abnormalities in spinocerebellar ataxias. In: Gazulla J, editor. Spinocerebellar Ataxias.

Rijeka: Intech; 2012. pp. 59-76. ISBN 979-953-307-095-6

[78] Seshagiri DV, Pal P, Jain S, Yadav R. Optokinetic nystagmus in SCA patients: A bedside test for oculomotor dysfunction grading. Neurology. 2018;**91**(13):e1255-e1261. DOI: 10.1212/WNL.0000000000006250

[79] Velazquez-Perez L, Seifried C, Abele M, Wirjatijasa F, Rodriguez-Labrada R, Santos-Falcon N, et al. Saccade velocity is reduced in presymptomatic spinocerebellar ataxia type 2. Clinical Neurophysiology. 2009;**120**:632-635. ISSN 1388-2457

[80] Velazquez-Perez L, Seifried C, Santos-Falcon N, Abele M, Ziemann U, Almaguer LE, et al. Saccade velocity is controlled by polyglutamine size in spinocerebellar ataxia 2. Annals of Neurology. 2004;**56**:444-447. ISSN 1531-8249

[81] Rodríguez-Labrada R, Vázquez-Mojena Y, Canales-Ochoa N, Medrano-Montero J, Velázquez-Pérez L. Heritability of saccadic eye movements in Spinocerebellar ataxia type 2: Insights into an endophenotype marker. Cerebellum & Ataxias. 2017;**19**:19

[82] Rodríguez-Labrada R, Velázquez-Pérez L, Auburger G, Ziemann U, Canales N, Medrano J, et al. Spinocerebellar ataxia type 2: Measures of saccade changes improve power for clinical trials. Movement Disorders. 2016;**31**:570-578

[83] Rodríguez-Labrada R, Velázquez-Pérez L, Seigfried C, et al. Saccadic latency is prolonged in spinocerebellar ataxia type 2 and correlates with the frontal-executive dysfunctions. Journal of the Neurological Sciences. 2011;**306**:106-107

[84] Rodríguez-Labrada R, Velázquez-Perez L, Seifried-Oberschmidt C,

Peña-Acosta A, Canales-Ochoa N, Medrano-Montero J, et al. Executive deficit in spinocerebellar ataxia type 2 is related to expanded CAG repeats: Evidence from antisaccadic eye movements. Brain and Cognition. 2014;**91**:28-34

[85] Velázquez-Pérez L, Rodríguez-Labrada R, Cruz-Rivas EM, et al. Comprehensive study of early features in spinocerebellar ataxia 2: Delineating the prodromal stage of the disease. Cerebellum. 2014;**13**:568-579

[86] Matilla-Dueñas A, Goold R, Giunti P. Clinical, genetic, molecular, and pathophysiological insights into spinocerebellar ataxia type 1. The Cerebellum. 2008;**7**:106-114. ISSN 1473-4222

[87] Klostermann W, Zuhlke C, Heide W, Kompf D, Wessel K. Slow saccades and other eye movement disorders in spinocerebellar atrophy type 1. Journal of Neurology. 1997;**244**:105-111. ISSN 0340-5354

[88] Jardim LB, Pereira ML, Silveira I, Ferro A, Sequeiros J, Giugliani R. Neurologic findings in Machado-Joseph disease: Relation with disease duration, subtypes, and (CAG)n. Archives of Neurology. 2011;**58**:899-904. ISSN 1538-3687

[89] Ghasia FF, Wilmot G, Ahmed A, Shaikh AG. Strabismus and micro-opsoclonus in Machado-Joseph disease. Cerebellum. 2016;**15**(4):491-497. DOI: 10.1007/ s12311-015-0718-0

[90] Wong SH, Patel L, Plant GT. Acquired esotropia in cerebellar disease: A case series illustrating misdiagnosis as isolated lateral rectus paresis and progression over time. Neuroophthalmology. 2015;**39**:59-63. DOI: 10.3109 01658107.2014.991832

[91] Colen C, Ketko A, George E, Van Stavern G. Periodic alternating nystagmus and periodic alternating skew deviation in spinocerebellar ataxia type 6. Journal of Neuro-Ophthalmology. 2008;**28**:287-288. ISSN 1536-5166

[92] Kim JM, Lee JY, Kim HJ, Kim JS, Kim YK, Park SS, et al. The wide clinical spectrum and nigrostriatal dopaminergic damage in spinocerebellar ataxia type 6. Journal of Neurology, Neurosurgery & Psychiatry. 2010;**81**:529-532. ISSN 1468-330X

[93] Christova P, Anderson JH, Gomez C. Impaired eye movements in presymptomatic spinocerebellar ataxia type 6. Archives of Neurology. 2008;**65**:530-536. ISSN 1538-3687

[94] Miller R, Tewari A, Miller J, Garbern J, Van Stavern GP. Neuro-ophthalmologic features of spinocerebellar ataxia type 7. Journal of Neuro-Ophthalmology. 2009;**29**: 180-186, ISSN 1536-5166

[95] Manrique RK, Noval S, Aguilar-Amat MJ, Arpa J, Rosa I, Contreras I. Ophthalmic features of spinocerebellar ataxia type 7. Journal of Neuro-Ophthalmology. 2009;**29**: 174-179, ISSN 1536-5166

[96] Oh AK, Jacobson KM, Jen JC, Baloh RW. Slowing of voluntary and involuntary saccades: An early sign in spinocerebellar ataxia type 7. Annals of Neurology. 2001;**49**:801-804. ISSN 1531-8249

[97] Hubner J, Sprenger A, Klein C, Hagenah J, Rambold H, Zuhlke C, et al. Eye movement abnormalities in spinocerebellar ataxia type 17 (SCA17). Neurology. 2007;**69**:1160-1168. ISSN 0028-3878

[98] Fahey MC, Cremer PD, Aw ST, Millist L, Todd MJ, White OB, et al. Vestibular, saccadic and fixation abnormalities in genetically confirmed Friedreich ataxia. Brain. 2008;**131** (Pt 4):35-45

[99] Hocking DR, Fielding J, Corben LA,
Cremer PD, Millist L, White OB,
et al. Ocular motor fixation deficits
in Friedreich ataxia. Cerebellum.
2010;**9**(3):411-418

[100] Fielding J, Corben L, Cremer
P, Millist L, White O, Delatycki
M. Disruption to higher order processes
in Friedreich ataxia. Neuropsychologia.
2010;**48**:235-242